HOW DO I KNOW IF I HAVE HPV?

Sometimes HPV-infected cells manifest themselves as genital warts. But other times the infection has no visible symptoms and only a Pap smear can tell if you have *precancerous disease of the cervix—or if you have cancer.*

ARE PAP SMEARS ACCURATE?

Most of the time. This essential reference spells out the do's and don'ts before your test, the new options that improve accuracy, and what the results of your Pap smear mean.

HOW DANGEROUS IS CERVICAL CANCER?

Before the invention of the Pap smear, it was the second leading cause of cancer death in women. Today, cervical cancer is *almost completely preventable.* That is why you need the facts about your risk level—and why you need regular Pap smears!

HOW CAN I TELL IF A PARTNER HAS HPV?

Some types of HPV can cause bumpy warts, but often penile HPV can only be found by a doctor—and symptom-free doesn't mean infection-free! Find out how he can infect—or re-infect—you!

WHAT YOUR DOCTOR MAY *NOT* TELL YOU ABOUT HPV AND ABNORMAL PAP SMEARS

WHAT YOUR DOCTOR MAY *NOT* TELL YOU ABOUT

HPV AND ABNORMAL PAP SMEARS

JOEL PALEFSKY, M.D., WITH JODY HANDLEY

WARNER BOOKS

An AOL Time Warner Company

This book is not intended as a substitute for medical advice of physicians. The reader should regularly consult a physician in all matters relating to his or her health, and particularly in respect of any symptoms that may require diagnosis or medical attention.

Copyright © 2002 by Dr. Joel Palefsky
All rights reserved.

Illustrations on pages: 13, 16, 20, 34, 220, and 295, by Ira C. Smith.

The title of the series What Your Doctor May *Not* Tell You About . . . and the related trade dress are trademarks owned by Warner Books, Inc., and may not be used without permission.

Warner Books, Inc., 1271 Avenue of the Americas, New York, NY 10020

Visit our Web site at www.twbookmark.com.

An AOL Time Warner Company

Printed in the United States of America

First Printing: May 2002

10 9 8 7 6 5 4 3 2

Library of Congress Cataloging-in-Publication Data

Palefsky, Joel.
    What your doctor may not tell you about HPV and abnormal pap smears / Joel Palefsky and Jody Handley.
        p. cm.
    Includes bibliographical references and index.
    ISBN 0-446-67787-6
    1. Papillomavirus diseases.   2. Pap test.   3. Cervix uteri—Cancer—Diagnosis.
I. Handley, Jody.   II. Title.
RC168.P15 P34 2002
616.69'25—dc21   2001056775

Book design and text composition by Charles A. Sutherland
Cover design by Diane Luger

This book is dedicated with love to Glenn, Raphael, my mother, and to the loving memory of my father.

ACKNOWLEDGMENTS

My thanks to the many researchers who preceded me in the study of Human Papillomavirus, and to my many colleagues who continue to lead the fight against anogenital cancer.

My thanks also to my wonderful laboratory and clinical staff for their hard work and dedication, and to Edwin Peacock for his technical assistance.

CONTENTS

AUTHOR'S NOTE: A Word on the Setup of this Book   xi

PART ONE:
What You Need to Know First   1

    CHAPTER ONE: HPV 101   3

    CHAPTER TWO: Pap Smears 101   51

PART TWO:
Cervical HPV   77

    CHAPTER THREE: Unsatisfactory, Normal, and
      Benign Pap Smears   79

    CHAPTER FOUR: Abnormal Paps: An ASCUS Diagnosis   95

    CHAPTER FIVE: Abnormal Paps: An LSIL Diagnosis   115

    CHAPTER SIX: Abnormal Paps: An HSIL Diagnosis   129

    CHAPTER SEVEN: Cervical Cancer   146

PART THREE:
Anogenital Dysplasias in Areas Other
Than the Cervix: Vagina, Vulva, and Anus   183

    CHAPTER EIGHT: Vaginal Dysplasia and Cancer   185

CHAPTER NINE: Vulvar Dysplasia and Cancer   203

CHAPTER TEN: Anal Dysplasia and Cancer   215

PART FOUR:
Benign HPV Infection   251

CHAPTER ELEVEN: GENITAL WARTS   253

CHAPTER TWELVE: Methods of Treatment
  for Genital Warts   266

CHAPTER THIRTEEN: Recurrent Respiratory
  Papillomatosis   279

PART FIVE:
Anal and Penile HPV Infections in Men   287

CHAPTER FOURTEEN: Men and HPV   289

PART SIX:
Taking Control   319

CHAPTER FIFTEEN: Living with HPV and Talking with
  Your Partner   321

PART SEVEN:
Hope for the Future   341

CHAPTER SIXTEEN: Looking Ahead   343

GLOSSARY   351
APPENDIX A: Choosing Your Gynecologist   363
APPENDIX B: Pelvic Self-Examination   365
APPENDIX C: Penile Self-Examination   368
APPENDIX D: Resources   370
REFERENCES   373
INDEX   385

Author's Note:
A Word on the Setup
of this Book

Over the years, my patients have repeatedly asked me, "What can I read?" and I've never had a good answer for them. There's plenty of medical literature on human papillomavirus (HPV) and the diseases that it causes, but relatively little out there for the general public (although some public sources that offer information about HPV are excellent, such as the American Social Health Association). But I felt that the time was right for a book on this subject—one that could be read and understood by people without a medical background.

Why now? Several reasons: HPV continues to spread, but people don't talk about it like they talk about other infections. In addition, recent developments in our understanding of how HPV causes cervical and other genital cancers, as well as the availability of better therapy, constitute important public information. Most important, people continue to die of HPV-related cancers, when, theoretically, they're all preventable!

Some numbers: In the United States, the yearly incidence of cervical cancer is about eight to ten per one hundred thousand women. That means that for every one hundred thousand women, eight to ten will develop cervical cancer every year. That probably doesn't sound like a lot to you, especially when compared to more common cancers such as breast cancer and colon cancer. But this number translates into about fourteen thousand new cases each year, and four thousand to five thousand women die of this preventable disease in the United States every year. Many more women will develop abnormalities on their cervix that could lead to cancer if left undiagnosed and untreated.

Pap smears are the first line of defense against cervical cancer. Another term commonly used for a Pap smear is *cervical cytology*. The word *cytology* means "study of cells," and the test allows your health care team to examine the cells of the cervix for signs of cancer or precancer. In countries around the world where women have no routine Pap smear screening, cervical cancer ranks as one of the most common causes of death among young women, as common as or more common than Human Immunodeficiency Virus infection. Other cancers related to HPV kill people as well: vulvar, vaginal, penile, and anal cancer. HPV can even cause cancer of the mouth. Some of these cancers, such as anal cancer, increase every year in the general population and in special high-risk populations. (We'll talk more about that later.) When was the last time you discussed anal cancer with your friends? Or your doctor?

Another fact: Most men and women who are sexually active will acquire a genital HPV infection at some point in their lives. Approximately 5.5 million new cases of sexually transmitted HPV will occur every year in the United States.

In fact, most will acquire HPV infection after having had sex with their first few sexual partners! Another important fact: HPV is spread by skin-to-skin contact, and while condoms may *reduce* the transmission of HPV, they do not completely *prevent* it.

I think it's time that HPV came out of the closet. People need to talk about it like they do any other medical issue. Women need to understand how they can get HPV and how HPV can cause potentially fatal diseases. They need to learn how to protect themselves. They need to learn how to play a more active role in their gynecological health care, and they need to learn the right questions to ask their doctors. In the summer of 2000, I had the privilege of attending the International AIDS Conference in Durban, South Africa. The theme of that conference was "Break the Silence." There was and is not enough discussion and education about HIV in South Africa and other countries, a silence that contributes to the spread of that virus. Sitting at this conference, I couldn't help but be struck by the silence that also surrounds HPV.

There are several reasons for this silence. Trying to get all the information from your doctor is sometimes difficult because nobody has enough time to really explain things properly. HPV is not a simple virus. And, in some cases, the doctors don't have enough information themselves, even if they have enough time. What about talking about HPV with your friends or peers? I'll bet it doesn't happen much either. Let's face it—anogenital warts, Pap smears, and cancer aren't exactly cocktail-party talk!

So this book is designed to fill these gaps and give you

the knowledge you'll need to make intelligent choices. I envision three audiences for this book:

One: women who have or have had an abnormal Pap smear and want to know its possible causes and ramifications.

Two: women and men who have or have had genital warts.

Three: women and men who are concerned about anogenital HPV infection and want to know more about it.

For organizational purposes, I'm starting off with part 1, "What You Need to Know First," which includes two crash courses. Chapter 1, "HPV 101," is an introduction to everything you need to know about HPV, the virus: the pathology, epidemiology, physiology, and all the other "ologies" scientists throw around. Chapter 2, "Pap Smears 101," is an explanation of how we interpret Pap smears and what they mean.

Part 2, "Cervical HPV," covers the oncogenic HPV types associated with cancer in the cervix as well as each different category of Pap smears, ranging from "unsatisfactory" to carcinoma. The word *oncogenic* means "causing cancer," and this is a term that I'll use often. This section of the book will include definitions, diagnostic procedures, and treatments for each condition.

Part 3, "Anogenital Dysplasias in Areas Other Than the Cervix," covers those other parts of the female anogenital region (the area that includes the anus and genitals) that can be affected by cancer-causing HPV types, such as the vulva, vagina, and anus.

Part 4, "Benign HPV Infection," covers the types of HPV that don't cause cancer, but can cause genital warts (cauliflowerlike lesions on the vulva, vagina, and anus) as well as a rare condition called recurrent respiratory papillomatosis.

Part 5, "Anal and Penile HPV Infections in Men," covers how both oncogenic and benign HPV types affect men, including penile and anal cancer and penile and anal warts.

Part 6, "Taking Control," offers some advice on how to live with HPV, how to talk to your sexual partners about HPV, and how to decrease the likelihood of further transmission.

Part 7, "Hope for the Future," includes some news about the development of new therapies for HPV infection and HPV-associated disease, including vaccinations against HPV.

Although HPV is not an issue that affects only women, for the reader's benefit early sections of this book are aimed primarily at women. As I said, several chapters offer advice on talking to your partner regarding oncogenic HPV and genital warts. In addition, chapters on penile and anal infection cover how some HPV types will affect a man's health and life. Men can suffer the consequences of HPV infection of the penis and anus—everything from warts to invasive cancer. Like women, men may experience considerable anxiety about anogenital HPV infection, not only because of fears for their own health, but also fear of spreading the virus to their partners.

Although most people think about HPV infection in the context of heterosexual relationships, and most of this book refers to women who have sex with men and vice versa, HPV affects just about anyone who is sexually active. In this book I include information for women who have sex with women (WSW) and men who have sex with men (MSM). Like other researchers, I prefer to use these purely descriptive terms because some WSW and MSM do not consider themselves to be "lesbian," "gay," or "homosexual."

You'll find two recurring themes throughout the book: One, the more you know, the more you'll understand your body; and two, with medical vigilance, a healthy body, and a healthy attitude, HPV will rarely lead to serious illness.

Finally, some of what you'll read in this book represents work done by my own research group, but it's a small fraction of the total. Most of the knowledge in this book is the product of many scientists and clinicians around the world who've dedicated their careers to the fight against HPV and anogenital cancer. While there are too many to mention individually, I gratefully acknowledge their contributions.

PART ONE

What You Need to Know First

CHAPTER ONE

HPV 101

The Facts

An estimated 75 percent of sexually active adults have or will have transmitted human papillomavirus (HPV) at some point in their lifetimes.

Over 75 percent of women have never even *heard* of HPV. It's important to understand that *HPV* should not be confused with *HIV*, which stands for "human immuno-deficiency virus." These two viruses are very different and affect women differently. That said, HPV and HIV can both infect women, and the interaction between these two viruses is discussed later in the book.

If it were up to me, the moment a woman came in for an annual gynecologic exam, she'd be told about HPV: the risk factors, the frequency, the consequences. Knowledge is power, says "Schoolhouse Rock," and I believe that knowledge leads to wiser, more informed choices. That's why I'm starting off this book with a crash course.

Why should you care about HPV? Because HPV is the most common sexually transmitted virus. HPV can be frightening, since not only do most women acquire it at some point, but it contributes to the development of pre-cancerous cervical disease (also known as *cervical dyspla-sia*, or *cervical intraepithelial neoplasia*) and cervical cancer. HPV, along with other factors, is the cause of dysplasia. But wait—there's more! HPV is versatile and also causes warts!

Your doctor may talk to you about Pap smears, warts, and dysplasia. So why don't doctors tell their patients about HPV? Probably a bunch of reasons. Perhaps they're embar-rassed to talk about sexually transmitted diseases (STDs), like many people are from time to time. A few doctors don't know much about HPV themselves. Maybe they don't even *know* the risks involved with HPV. Others don't bother saying anything about HPV because there's no treat-ment for the virus itself, only treatment for the diseases the virus causes (such as warts, precancerous lesions of the cervix, and cervical cancer). They're all reasons why *you* may have to bring up the subject with your doctor if he or she doesn't. (You'll notice that I use the word *doctor* in this book. However, a wide range of health professionals actu-ally provide many of the services referred to in the book, including nurses, nurse practitioners, and physician's assis-tants. So if one of these other health professionals is in-volved in your care, you can substitute them for *doctor* as appropriate.)

From your perspective, discussing STDs could be diffi-cult as well. Many health professionals have difficulty leaving their own personal prejudices and judgments at the door, so you may feel as though Dr. Smith is condemning you when she says the risk of HPV increases with the number of sexual partners. Indeed, though she's telling the truth—your sexual behavior *does* affect the chances of getting any STD—her tone may suggest condemnation, disappointment, arrogance, or condescension.

The real issue, after all, is not your past behavior. You can't change that and Dr. Smith can't change that. What you *can* control is your health and practices in the present and future, and even there, I've heard horror stories from patients.

"I had a friend with HPV, so when my doctor told me I had it, I knew how to handle it and what it meant," said Karen, twenty-seven. "*Then* he told me that everyone on the street probably had it, so I didn't have to tell my partner!"

Why would you tell your patient that her partner doesn't need to know she has a sexually transmitted virus? Especially when *he* might have been the one who gave it to her?

Your past choices, whether or not you regret them now, are unchangeable. If you didn't know your partner had HPV—indeed, maybe *he* didn't know—then that's unfortunate . . . and also in the past. Now, you have the power to monitor your health, keep the HPV under control, make more educated choices about your sexual practices, and inform your partners so *they* can make more educated choices. With the knowledge in this book, you're armed with information that can save your life and other people's lives. *You have the power.*

Now that you know why I think you need to know this information, let's get started.

HPV: Bare-Bones Basics

First and foremost, I want you to understand that HPV only infects the skin, and the term in medicalese for skin is *epithelium*. The skin, or epithelium, lines not only our whole body, but also inside some of our internal organs.

HPV only infects the epithelium: the skin lining the outside *and* inside of some of your internal organs.

Because of this particular trait, the only diseases caused by HPV are those of the skin. The skin is our coat of armor; it protects us from the environment and keeps us healthy. We have two kinds of skin: *cutaneous* and *mucosal.*

Cutaneous skin surfaces are what you usually think of as "skin": the dry, occasionally hairy skin on your arms and legs. This kind of skin has a thick protective coating called *keratin.*

Mucosal skin surfaces, known as *mucous membranes,* are the wet ones: your mouth, vagina, and anus. These also contain keratin, but the protective coating is much thinner.

More than one hundred types of HPV infect humans. Like the skin, they're divided into two subgroups: those that infect cutaneous skin and those that infect mucosal skin. (HPVs are numbered 1, 2, 3, etc., much like hepatitis is lettered A, B, C, and so on.) Both types of HPV, cutaneous and mucosal, are spread through surface contact: from skin to skin, or mucous membrane to mucous membrane, or skin to mucous membrane, or mucous membrane to skin. . . . Imagine the possibilities! But since HPVs infect only the skin, they do *not* cause disease in other organs like the blood, bones, liver, heart (unless the skin cells infected with HPV spread to those organs in a process called *metastasis*, which I'll talk about later). Also, HPVs can't be acquired through a blood transfusion.

Cutaneous HPVs mostly cause warts on your skin— they're infectious and tenacious. (By the way, you *don't* get warts from toads! Lots of animals have their own papilloma viruses—rabbits, cows, dogs, to name a few. All papilloma viruses are extremely species specific and cannot be passed between species. So you can't get them by touching animals.)

HPV is particular in other ways. Not only does it only hang out in its own species (humans), but each of the more than one hundred HPV types has its own favorite hangout in the skin of the human body. Some HPV types prefer the cutaneous skin, and some prefer the mucosal skin. Some like the hands and feet, and some like the genital region. They rarely, if ever, cross over!

The most common skin HPV types are HPV 1, 2, and 4, and these cause warts on the hands (palmar warts) and feet (plantar warts). Almost all of us have had warts on the hands or feet at some time. Fortunately, HPV 1, 2, and 4 don't like to live in the skin of the genital tract, so these HPV types rarely—if ever—cause genital warts, precancerous genital lesions, or cancer. This means that you *can-*

not get these lesions by touching the hands or feet of another person.

On the other hand, a group of HPV types do prefer the cutaneous and mucosal skin of the genital region. These HPV types *can* cause warts, precancerous lesions, or cancer in your genital area. As I mentioned earlier, the HPV types that are associated with cancer are called oncogenic. They're sometimes also called *intermediate-risk* or *high-risk* HPV types. The HPV types not associated with cancer—typically the ones that cause warts—are called *nononcogenic, benign,* or *low-risk* HPV types. The most common cancer-causing genital HPV types are HPV 16 and HPV 18, while the most common low-risk HPV types are HPV 6 and 11. While most of the thirty to forty known types of mucosal HPVs typically infect your genital tract, a few, such as HPV 13 and HPV 32, prefer the mucous membranes of the mouth.

Here's an important point about the skin-site preferences of the various HPV types. Since the genital HPV types live only in the genital skin, and since HPV is spread by skin-to-skin contact, then it seems as though most, if not all, genital HPV infection is *sexually* transmitted: It spreads by one person's genitalia touching another person's genitalia. Remember—the genital HPV types live only in the genital skin, and not in the other parts of your skin, such as your hands, face, and so on. So you can't get a genital HPV infection by touching the hand or foot of someone with warts in those places. To acquire a genital HPV infection, there usually needs to be genital-to-genital skin contact. Having said that, there *are* some other methods of sexual transmission, and I'll talk about them later.

Risk Category	HPV Type	Oncogenic Risk	Comments
Low	6, 11	Rarely found in cervical cancer	These types most commonly cause g...ui waris, covered in part 3 of this book.
Intermediate	33, 35, 39, 51, 52, 56, 58, 59, 68	Found in about 25% of cervical cancers	Although these types may be oncogenic, they're rarer than the high-risk types.
High	16, 18, 31, 45	Found in about 75% of cervical cancers	Types 16 and 18 are the most common of the high-risk types.

*Source: K V. Shah, "What Are Human Papillomaviruses?" (paper presented at the Eighteenth International Papillomavirus Conference and HPV Clinical Workshop jointly with the Twelfth Meeting of the Spanish Association of Cervical Pathology and Colposcopy, Barcelona, Spain, July 2000).

Not all mucosal HPV types cause cancer, though. The chart above displays the cervical cancer risk of genital HPV types. Keep in mind, though, that "intermediate" risk doesn't mean those types won't cause cancer; it only means that they're found in fewer cancers. If you have an intermediate type, your risk of developing cancer may be similar to high-risk types.

Genital warts are caused by HPV types 6 and 11. These are the cauliflowerlike lesions, similar to other warts on your body, that can be found anywhere in the genital tract, including the anus, vulva, vagina, or penis. They're also nononcogenic—they won't cause cancer. But they're a pain, to be sure! I'll cover HPV 6 and 11 in great detail in part 4 of this book.

High or intermediate risk, or oncogenic, types don't always cause visible lesions, but they *do* cause cancer. In fact, *99 percent of all cervical cancers have been linked to oncogenic HPV types.*

A Quick History

Before George Papanicolaou invented the Pap smear in the 1940s, cervical cancer caused the deaths of more women, worldwide, than any other type of cancer. I've had patients whose grandmothers, great-aunts, probably even great-grandmothers died of cervical cancer. Eva Perón, the famed Evita, wife of Juan Perón of Argentina, died of cervical cancer—and so did Juan Perón's first wife, which might indicate that all three of them had HPV. It's only been in the last fifteen years or so that we've made the connection between HPV and cervical cancer, and sexual transmission was not proven until 1954, a decade after the Pap smear was first instituted. Genital warts, caused by different types of HPV than those that cause cancer, were recognized in antiquity, all the way back to second-century Soranus's chapter entitled "On Warty Excrescences of the Female Genitalia" (Campion 1996).

I'd like to share a quote with you, one I really like. In his section from the series Treatise of Venereal Diseases in Nine Books from 1737, entitled "Of Porri, Verrucae and Condylomata of the Pudenda," John Astruc wrote, "There remains a fourth species of venereal diseases to be added to those which we have already described, viz warty excresences of the genitals which succeed impure coition, but for the most part, follow other pocky disorders that have been ill managed. Sometimes they wither of themselves and fall off, leaving a root behind them, from which they spring up afresh; sometimes they are permanent, but are flaccid, soft, and almost void of sense; sometimes hard, dry, rigid, horny, destitute of sense and perfectly callous; but sometimes they are painful, having an ichorous discharge from their heads, and seem to be of a *cancerous* nature."

This quotation, graphic though it may be, summarizes so much of what we know about warts and anogenital cancer: They're sexually acquired (*coition* is an old term for sex), difficult to get rid of, and have a variety of appearances, and perhaps most important, warts are somehow related to cancer. Back in 1737, they didn't know that the common link between warts and cancer was HPV. In fact, we didn't know it until about fifteen years ago! Despite this new realization, it's clear that HPV is not a new virus and that cancers and warts caused by HPV aren't new diseases. They'll likely continue to be around for a long, long time, unless we can eradicate HPV with a vaccine. (See part 7.)

Virology and HPV 101

As you know, HPV is a virus, and viruses are tiny, infectious parasites that thrive and reproduce within living cells. They need to live in human cells and cannot live outside human cells by themselves. Some scientists speculate that viruses are among the oldest "living" organisms, if one can call them that.

Usually, a virus consists of a protein shell, or *capsid*, enclosing a nucleic acid, either *deoxyribonucleic acid (DNA)* or *ribonucleic acid (RNA)*. The capsid is the protective

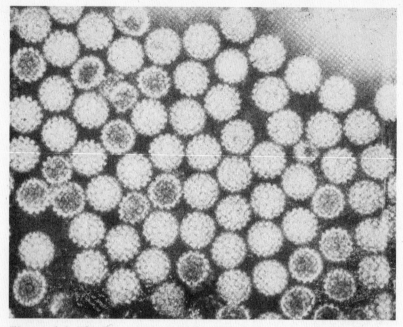

Figure 1.1: Electron Micrograph of HPV Particles. *This figure shows what the mature HPV particles actually look like in a cell as seen through a special instrument called an electron microscope. The viral particles are comprised of the L1 and L2 proteins, but mostly L1. (Reprinted by permission of Pearson Education, Inc., Upper Saddle River, NJ 07458.)*

coating of the virus. (A picture of HPV capsids as they appear under an electron microscope is shown in fig. 1.1.) The DNA of an organism, such as a human or a virus, is collectively called its *genome*. The DNA in the genome is organized into units known as *genes*. Collectively, the *genes* in our genome contain all the information we need to live and reproduce (after all, reproduction is one of nature's primary goals).

HPVs are double-stranded DNA viruses, which means that they're made up of two DNA strands (much like human

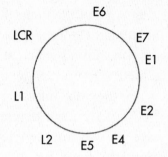

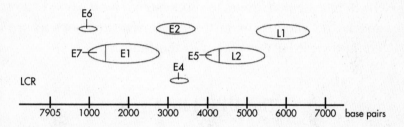

Figure 1.2: HPV Genome. *This picture shows the organization of the HPV genome. The DNA of the virus lives in cells as a circle that divides when the cell divides. The virus genome contains the code for six early proteins, denoted with an "E" for "early." These are called early because thay are among the first to be produced in a cell after infection. The E6 and E7 proteins are the HPV proteins most responsible for development of cancer. Proteins produced later in the life cycle of the virus are denoted with an "L" for "late." The L1 and L2 proteins make up the HPV viral capsid, or protective coating, that surrounds the viral DNA in a mature, infectious viral particle. (Illustration by Ira C. Smith.)*

DNA). The DNA in each gene gives instructions to the cell on how to make proteins, which in turn are made of molecules called *amino acids*. Proteins are the workhorses of the cells: They do everything for the cell, from digesting its food to cleaning up its messes. Humans have hundreds of thousands of genes, and many of these were only recently identified when the DNA sequence of the entire human genome was determined in the Human Genome Project.

HPV has a genome, too, but it's much smaller than the human genome. In fact, HPV 16 and 18 get away with having only eight genes, since they use human genes for much of their dirty work. (See fig. 1.2 for a diagram of the HPV genome.) Scientists have known the complete genome sequence of many different HPV types for about fifteen years, which has helped them to understand how HPV causes cancer, and allowed them to design new strategies to prevent and treat HPV infection in the future.

The HPV Life Cycle

Infection with HPV occurs when HPV enters the anogenital skin, or epithelium. Understanding how the epithelium works is important to understanding what HPV does, so I'll explain a bit about your "protective coating." As we said earlier, the skin is your coat of armor. It actually consists of several layers of epithelial cells that sit on a structure called the *basement membrane*. Below the basement membrane is a mixture of compounds and cells collectively known as the *stroma*. (See fig. 1.3 for a diagram of the cervical epithelium.)

The skin is a continuously renewing organ. Skin cells from the surface continually die and fall off (that's what you wash off your face every day, and that's what dandruff is). With surface cells dying and falling off all the time, how do you continue to have skin? It's because you also have cells at the bottom whose sole purpose is to keep making more surface cells. In medicalese, we say the epithelium is constantly "turning over."

Those cells at the bottom are long-living cells called *basal cells*. They sit directly on the basement membrane, and their function is to keep dividing. By continuing to divide, they constantly generate new skin. The basal cells live so long they're almost immortal. As they divide, their daughter cells (if you're a woman) or son cells (if you're a man) get pushed up into the upper layers of the epithelium, and as they do, they mature. When they mature, they change shape and create some of the keratin that provides an extra-protective coating on the surface. Finally, after about thirty days, they reach the top of the epithelium and fall off like generations before.

Then the whole cycle begins again. Basically, each basal cell divides and pushes its children, grandchildren, great-grandchildren, and so on, into the wide world of skin, where eventually they'll end their short lives in about a month.

Why am I telling you all this? To establish infection, HPV must first infect these immortal basal cells. This has important implications for the course of HPV infection, and for why HPV infection is so difficult to eradicate and treat.

The first implication is that HPV must first run a gauntlet of several cell layers before it can reach the basal cells, its preferred target. Simple exposure of the surface of the skin to HPV particles or HPV DNA probably isn't enough to lead to infection. However, minor trauma to the epithelium, as might occur during sex, is enough to allow viral particles to break through to the basal cell layer. But depending on

Low-grade squamous intraepithelial lesion (LSIL)		High-grade squamous intraepithelial lesion (HSIL)	
Condyloma	CIN grade 1	CIN grade 2	CIN grade 3
Normal	Very mild to mild dysplasia	Moderate dysplasia	Severe dysplasia / In situ carcinoma

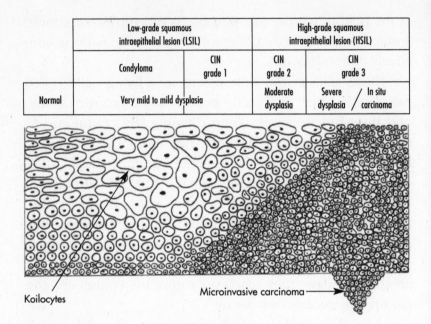

Koilocytes

Microinvasive carcinoma ────▶

Figure 1.3: Cervical Epithelium Ranging from Normal to Invasive Cancer. *This figure shows what the normal epithelium looks like on the left. The terminology used to describe the abnormal areas, or "lesions," is shown on the top of the diagram. Progressively more advanced changes in the epithelium due to HPV are shown as the diagram moves to the right. Epithelial cells sit on a structure called the basement membrane. The normal epithelium shows cells flattening out and losing their nucleus as they mature and move up to the top of the epithelium. These cells eventually die and fall off. Mild dysplasia is characterized by relatively minor changes in the cells and sometimes by the presence of koilocytes, which are cells with enlarged, irregular nuclei surrounded by a halo. Mild dysplasia does not directly progress to cancer. Moderate and severe dysplasia occur when an increasing proportion of the normal epithelium is replaced by small cells with large nuclei. The most advanced form of severe dysplasia is known as* carcinoma in situ, *in which the entire epithelium is replaced by these cells. Severe dysplasia can progress to cancer, which by definition occurs once the epithelial cells invade the basement membrane and the underlying tissues. (Illustration by Ira C. Smith.)*

the number of minor traumas during sex and how often your partner's HPV comes in contact with your basal cells, infection can begin in many different basal cells. Remember, though, that trauma isn't even absolutely necessary for HPV to get down to the basal layer.

The second implication is that since HPV infects long-lived or immortal cells, HPV infection may also be long-lived. When the infected basal cells divide, so does the virus, and copies of the HPV genome go into each of the daughter or son cells. So, these basal cells may actually serve as a long-lived reservoir of HPV infection. Most of the information we have suggests that tests to detect HPV infection become negative over time in most women. But it's possible that we never truly rid ourselves of HPV. If so, HPV infection might be like herpes virus infection, which never goes away. This remains a controversial issue, but it's important to understand that in the vast majority of women, even if HPV persists for life, this kind of dormant infection causes no problems whatsoever. The typical patient is the woman who may have had HPV fifteen years ago, was treated for dysplasia, and has never shown a sign of an abnormal Pap since. If we were to use a test to detect HPV DNA in her cervix, we wouldn't find it. As figure 1.4 shows, most women over the age of thirty show neither HPV infection nor dysplasia—most of the HPV action is in the "under-thirty" set. Often, though, when a woman over the age of thirty has an organ transplant, her doctor puts her on immunosuppressing drugs to prevent rejection of the new organ. Once her body's immunity is compromised, she redevelops dysplasia and evidence of HPV infection. Another common example of this kind of thing is an

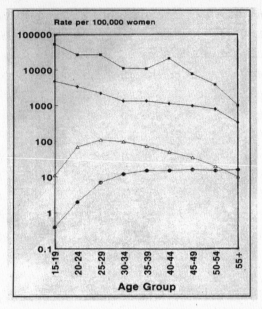

Figure 1.4: Age-Related Prevalence of HPV Infection, Dysplasia, and Invasive Cervical Cancer. *This figure shows the prevalence of cervical HPV infection, mild dysplasia, moderate to severe dysplasia, and invasive cervical cancer in five-year age groups. The scale on the left is a log scale showing the rates per 100,000 women. The line showing the prevalence of HPV infection (black squares) indicates that the highest prevalence of HPV infection is seen in young women under the age of twenty-four years and that a high proportion of women in this group have HPV. The prevalence declines thereafter, and most women over the age of thirty do not have detectable HPV infection. The line showing mild dysplasia (black diamonds) shows that a smaller proportion of women have mild dysplasia than have HPV infection, and that the peak prevalence is also less than twenty-four years. The line showing moderate to severe dysplasia (white triangles) indicates that an even smaller proportion of women have this more advanced form of dysplasia, and that the prevalence of moderate to severe dysplasia peaks in the twenty-five-to-twenty-nine-year-old age group. The line showing invasive cervical cancer (black circles) shows that only a very small proportion of women will develop cervical cancer and that the peak age prevalence is after the age of thirty-five years. (Illustration reprinted from Schiffman, M. H. "Recent Progress in Defining the Epidemiology of Human Papillomavirus Infection and Cervical Neoplasia." Journal of the National Cancer Institute 84 (1992) (6): 394–398 by permission of the Oxford University Press.)*

HIV-positive woman who may not have had evidence of abnormal Pap smears for much of her sexually active life, but once HIV starts to mess up her immune system, she develops dysplasia.

Was either of these women "reinfected?" Probably not. The recurrence of dysplasia, to me, indicates that HPV was dormant in her body during those years. Her healthy immune system kept it at bay. It's kind of like arthritis pain— many people experience it only when it's damp outside. Immunity suppressants, HIV infection, pregnancy—all of these factors can lead to dysplasia long after the fact, which suggests that HPV lives on in your system in small, dormant numbers.

I do want to stress, though, that this idea is hotly debated in the field—some researchers do believe that HPV can be definitively eradicated. Regardless, as I said before, even if small pockets of HPV do remain for life, in the vast majority of women it won't cause problems as they get older. I'll be covering the HIV question in detail in part 5, so for organizational purposes, we'll stick to HPV right now.

While HPV likes the basal cell layers of the epithelium, it's actually a bit pickier than that. It has a favorite kind of basal cell, located in a special area of the cervix known as the *transformation zone*. (This is shown in fig. 1.5.) The transformation zone, also known as the transition zone or TZ, is where the *endocervical columnar epithelium* meets the *exocervical squamous epithelium*. Got that? Basically, the top layer of the cervix—the epithelium—is further divided into two areas. The endocervical part lines the canal leading up to the uterus and produces your cervical mu-

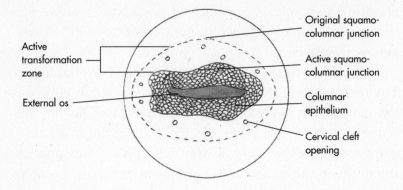

Figure 1.5: Cervix Showing the Transformation Zone. *This diagram shows the cervix as it might be seen looking through a vaginal speculum. The transformation zone, within the dotted line, is where the columnar cells of the endocervix meet the squamous cells of the endocervix. Most HPV infections, dysplasias, and cancers arise in this region of the cervix. (Illustration by Ira C. Smith.)*

cus. The exocervical part lines the outer part of the cervix. The area between them is called the transition, or transformation, zone. Since the TZ is the best place for HPV to infect the cervix, this is also where most of the HPV-associated cervical diseases arise, including cervical cancer.

After exposure to the basal cells and infection, the HPV life cycle begins. What happens at this point varies from person to person. Once the basal layer is penetrated, HPV loses its protein capsid. It crosses into the cell nucleus, where it can direct the cell to create some of its own proteins, and where the viral genome can reproduce itself. In some women, the virus just hangs out and doesn't do anything. It doesn't make any viral proteins and doesn't cause any obvious problems. In medicalese, the virus is *dormant* or *latent*.

On the other hand, in some women the virus becomes active immediately. In this situation, the virus not only makes a lot of proteins that cause changes in the epithelial cells, but they also make more HPV particles. Although the virus must first establish itself in the basal cell layer, most of the action is in the layers of more mature cells closer to the top, where the viral particles are actually produced. When the cells die and fall off the top layers, they probably release infectious HPV particles with them. Think of the basal cells as the "queen bee," while the daughter cells are "worker bees." The queen bee is almost immortal, but she stays in the hive all day, producing more little bees. It's the worker bees who go out and pollinate.

Why is the virus dormant in some women and active in others? That's an important question, and we don't have a complete answer for it. Several factors are probably involved. Some relate to the particular HPV type. Others relate to you as the host or hostess of the virus. As we've already learned, HPVs aren't all alike, and some are more aggressive than others. Scientists have also learned recently that even among a given HPV type such as the oncogenic, or cancer-causing HPV 16, some variants of it are worse than others. So here we have a luck of the draw—if you're exposed to HPV, you hope that it'll be a nononcogenic, or low-risk, HPV type. If you do get a cancer-causing type, you hope to be infected with one of the less aggressive kinds of that HPV type.

What about factors related to *you*? One of the most important is your genetic background, which determines how strong your immune response is to the virus. This may explain why some people are at a higher risk of developing cervical cancer even when they've been exposed to the same HPV type and variant. Smoking is a risk factor, and another important factor is your stress level: Higher stress levels weaken the immune system. Diet may also be important, since women with diets high in vegetables, fruit, carotenoids, and vitamins C and E may be at lower risk of developing cervical cancer. Some of these factors are in your control and some aren't. Although it's clearly important to have a good diet and be in overall good health, dysplasia or cancer can develop even in the healthiest of women. The bottom line? In most women, we don't know why HPV acts more aggressively than in others.

In summary, it may not be completely possible to influence the course of HPV infection, but some factors *are* within your control, relatively speaking. My prescription? Lower your stress levels, eat well, and stop smoking. Easy, right? Following this prescription will improve your overall health and may improve your chances against the virus. On the other hand, the virus may remain active even if you do everything you possibly can, and in this case, your best bet is to *continue* doing everything you can to remain healthy, and return for all of your follow-up visits with your doctor.

I've Been Exposed to HPV
What Happens Next?

As I said earlier, in many women, nothing will happen, and they won't even know they've been infected.

Incubation periods can last from two weeks to eight months or more, with an average of three months. At this point, your immune system is working to keep the infection at bay, although factors like the ones I listed above—genetic predisposition, smoking, nutrition—will contribute to the effectiveness of your immune response.

Incubation periods can also be indefinite; you could be exposed to HPV and not develop dysplasia for years, until your immunity is compromised in some way. In other women, HPV becomes active early on and results in a variety of epithelial changes. Most of these are not dangerous, but some could lead to cancer.

How Does HPV Cause Cervical Disease?

During active expression, the HPV-infected cells will begin to change. These cells will divide and multiply, creating more HPV-infected cells. These changes will either manifest as a clinically obvious disease such as warts or show as *subclinical* infection, which is as common or more common than clinical infection. Subclinical infections cannot be seen with the naked eye, but are only visible using special diagnostic procedures discussed later in this book.

Actual warts in your cervix, called *condyloma acuminata*, fall in the "genital wart" category and are usually caused by non-cancer-causing HPV types such as HPV 6 or 11. For organizational purposes, I'll be covering warts and HPV types 6 and 11 in part 4 of this book, but keep in mind that having types 6 or 11 doesn't rule out the possibility of also having HPV 16 or 18, the most common oncogenic types. HPV 16 and 18, like the other cancer-causing HPV types, produce cervical cancer and subclinical disease in the form of dysplasia. I'm going to have a lot more to say about dysplasia throughout this book.

In the basal cell layer, HPV generally doesn't do much, other than concentrate on reproducing its own genome so that more copies are available when the cell divides. There's relatively little or no activity in these cells, and few HPV proteins are being made, which may be how HPV persists in basal cells for long periods (maybe even for life). Most researchers believe that the body can clear HPV infection through development of an immune response to the virus. The immune system recognizes foreign protein, not the presence of the virus itself; if HPV doesn't produce these proteins in the basal cells, then your immune system won't detect anything unusual and will not respond.

Once the basal cells divide and push their children up into the cold, hard world of the maturing epithelium, it's a different story. All of the cells born of that basal cell form a kind of column, and if the basal cell was infected with HPV, all of its children will also be infected. However, once the cells begin to mature, the virus often activates. It produces the proteins necessary to make mature viral particles. So despite the fact that initial HPV infection occurs in the basal cell layer, most of the virus action occurs in the basal

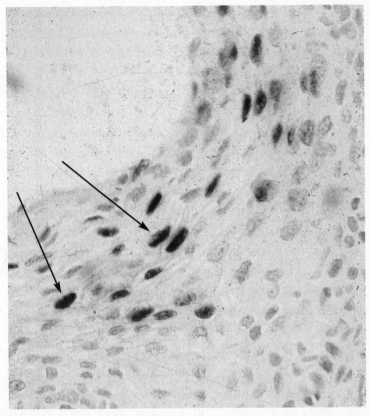

Figure 1.6: Biopsy of Mild-Dysplasia–Producing HPV DNA. *This figure shows a biopsy of mild dysplasia of the cervix, tested for the presence of HPV DNA, which is indicated by the presence of a dark stain in the nucleus of an infected cell (shown with the arrows). The figure shows that most of the virus DNA is present in the more mature cell layers. (Author's photo.)*

cells' children as they mature and move up through the epithelium.

The production of mature viral particles damages the cells, and one result of virus production is a change in the cells called *koilocytosis*, which occurs when koilocytes accumulate. The word *koilos* means "halo" in Greek, and a koilocyte is an epithelial cell, usually found in the surface layers, which has an enlarged, irregular cell nucleus surrounded by a halo or clear space. When properly diagnosed, koilocytosis is synonymous with HPV infection and active viral reproduction. When the virus actively reproduces and generates koilocytes, other changes in the skin may occur as well. The epithelial cells pile up on each other, producing a growth that you know as a wart. On the outer genitalia, you can feel these with your finger, or you know you have them because they itch, burn, or bleed. You probably won't even know that they're there if they're really high up in the genital tract, such as on the cervix. I'll have a lot more information for you about warts later in this book, but at this point it's worth knowing that warts are a major nuisance. However, they don't usually lead to cancer and so they literally won't kill you.

HPV thrives in the more mature, differentiated cells. Once the initial infection works its way to the topmost superficial layer, the virus multiplies like crazy, producing more DNA, more cells, and forming more viral particles. (Fig. 1.6 shows HPV DNA in the more mature layers of the cervical epithelium.) The sheer amount of viral DNA production leads many doctors to believe that having a wart is the most contagious stage of HPV infection. The more HPV particles floating around, the more likely they are to latch on to a cell and infect it—whether it's in the host's body or in the host's sexual partner.

Terminology 101

At this point, I need to introduce the many different terms that you'll need to understand. Below is a basic chart of the four classification systems that have been used over the years. Before we get to it, though, I need to explain the difference between a Pap smear and a biopsy (tissue sample). A Pap smear consists of a random sampling of cells that are taken from the surface of your cervix and placed at random on a slide or in a jar of solution. It's a sample of cells. If your doctor sees something wrong on the Pap smear, he or she can't tell where the abnormal cells came from. So the next step in your evaluation is to examine the cervix for the source of those cells. To confirm the abnormality, your doctor will cut off a small piece of the suspicious area to examine under a microscope. The sample of tissue obtained by the doctor is known as a *biopsy*, and that's what determines your treatment. To understand what the changes in the cervical tissue might look like, you can refer back to figure 1.3.

Why am I telling you this? The important thing to remember is that the "class" system and "Bethesda" system on the left of the chart on the next page refer primarily to grading Pap smears. Methods of classifying Pap smears have gone through several shifts since the Pap smear's invention. With new technologies, cytotechnologists and cytopathologists—the folks who examine and diagnose your Pap—can see more levels of change and can therefore assign more specific names to each level. That's why the Bethesda system largely replaced the class system. On the other hand, the "dysplasia" system and "CIN" system refer primarily to

Class System Rating (Pap Smears)	Bethesda System Rating (Pap Smears)	Dysplasia System Rating (Tissue Biopsies)	CIN (Cervical Intraepithelial Neoplasia) System Rating (Tissue Biopsies)	HPV Relationship Rating
0	Unsatisfactory	Unsatisfactory	Unsatisfactory	Not enough evidence to say
1	Within normal limits	Negative	Negative	−
1	Benign cellular changes	Negative	Negative	−
2	ASC-US[1] or AGUS[2] favor reactive	No term	No term	+/−
2	ASC-H[3] or AGUS favor neoplasia	No term	No term	+/−
3	LSIL[4]	Mild	CIN 1	+
3	HSIL[5]	Moderate	CIN 2	+
3	HSIL	Severe	CIN 3	+
4	HSIL	CIS (carcinoma in situ)	CIN 3	+
5	Carcinoma	Carcinoma	Carcinoma	+

[1]ASC-US = atypical squamous cells of undetermined significance
[2]AGUS = atypical glandular cells of undetermined significance
[3]ASC-H = atypical squamous cells; cannot exclude HSIL
[4]LSIL = low-grade squamous intraepithelial lesions
[5]HSIL = high-grade squamous intraepithelial lesions

cervical tissues as seen in a biopsy. The fifth column indicates that category's relationship to HPV. A "−" shows that it's not directly linked to HPV; a "+" indicates that it is directly linked to HPV; and a "+/−" shows that it may or may not be linked to HPV infection.

As you've probably guessed, the terminology describing changes in the cervix can be confusing and seems to change on a regular basis. Biopsies span a range of changes, and they're fairly self-explanatory, once you know what the acronyms mean. The mildest end of the spectrum includes mild dysplasia, also known as CIN 1. In biopsies, more advanced disease is classified as moderate (CIN 2) or severe dysplasia (CIN 3).

In Pap smears, different terminology is used, but there's a relationship between the Pap smear terms and the biopsy terms. In classifying Pap smears the term *squamous intraepithelial lesions* (SIL) is used. Low-grade SIL, or LSIL for short, is the Pap smear equivalent of mild dysplasia or CIN 1. In Pap smears, high-grade SIL, or HSIL for short, is the equivalent of both moderate *and* severe dysplasia. Got all that? There are, of course, other subtle differences in how these mostly equivalent terms are used. I'll explain these terms again later. But from now on, when I'm talking about tissues and biopsies, I'll use *dysplasia*. When I'm talking about Pap smears, I'll use *SIL*.

Here's why distinguishing moderate and severe dysplasia from mild dysplasia is so important: Mild dysplasia isn't considered to be precancerous and usually regresses by itself without treatment.

On the other hand, moderate and severe dysplasia—especially severe—could progress to cancer and needs to be diagnosed and treated before this can occur. By definition, invasive cancer is diagnosed when the cells of the cervix invade the basement membrane and enter the tissues below (fig. 1.3). It's also important to remember that some cases of mild dysplasia can progress to moderate or severe, and mild dysplasia must be watched carefully to ensure that it does regress. If it doesn't, then it usually needs treatment because it may progress to moderate or severe dysplasia.

What Are Moderate and Severe Dysplasia, and How Does HPV Cause Them?

Unlike mild dysplasia, which is the clinical manifestation of active HPV reproduction and mature virus particle formation, relatively few virus particles form in moderate and severe dysplasia. For this reason, you're probably more infectious when you have mild dysplasia than when the dysplasia is moderate or severe. Instead, in moderate or severe dysplasia, two HPV proteins (known as E6 and E7) encourage the cells to continue dividing, causing changes that are different from those of mild dysplasia (see fig. 1.2 and 1.3). While mild dysplasia may show the presence of koilocytes, the cells are not mutating so much—very little abnormal cell division occurs.

On the other hand, moderate and severe dysplasias are characterized by the replacement of more and more of the normal maturing epithelium with small, immature-looking cells. These cells look like the basal cells, but in moderate and severe dysplasia they're also found in the higher cell layers and sometimes reach all the way to the top. In moderate dysplasia, about half of the normal top layer of the cervix is replaced by these abnormal cells, and in severe dysplasia, they replace most, if not all, of the normal top layer. In severe dysplasia, the cervical cells divide all the way to the top layers, while in normal epithelium, cells divide only at the bottom.

The change from mild dysplasia to moderate or severe is critical: While mild dysplasia is not dangerous, moderate and severe dysplasia (especially severe) are potentially precancerous, and detection and treatment of moderate and severe dysplasia can prevent cervical cancer. Because severe dysplasia shows more advanced changes than moderate, the risk of progressing to invasive cancer from severe dysplasia is probably higher than that of moderate.

I should mention a few important points: First, not all women who develop dysplasia will develop cancer. Second, if it progresses at all, the time it takes to get from dysplasia to cancer is highly variable. In rare cases, it could take a few months; more commonly, it takes several years or even decades.

The mild-to-moderate-to-severe-to-invasive cancer processes are poorly understood. Some researchers believe that damage to your own genes (mutations) may drive the process forward, and that HPV plays a role by making your cells more susceptible to this genetic damage. (This is explained in greater detail in the next section.) Regardless of how this happens, once the cells reach a point of no return, they begin to divide uncontrollably. The rapidly growing cells may penetrate deep into the tissues under the basement membrane: the stroma. The cancer may eventually kill the woman by invading and destroying some of the vital organs in the pelvis or by spreading to distant parts of the body where they can interfere with organs such as the lung.

How HPV Does Its Dysplasia- and Cancer-Causing Dirty Work

Like all living things, a virus's primary job is to reproduce. A DNA virus like HPV must do two things to reproduce: (1) create more viral DNA to divide and create more viruses; and (2) keep its host alive so it can continue reproducing.

The cancer-causing HPV types, of course, sometimes fail to keep their host alive. This is probably a mistake of nature. Of the various genes encoded in the HPV genome, two genes—E6 and E7—are responsible for most of the cancer-causing potential. The E6 and E7 proteins bind to, and inactivate, the p53 and pRB cellular proteins, respectively the "guardians of the cell cycle" (Shah 2000).

How does the inactivation of the p53 and pRB proteins lead to cancer? Hang on, folks—this is a complex question with a complex answer!

A diagram showing how this might happen is shown in figure 1.7. Think of what a basal cell does in the course of its lifetime. On the one hand, it reproduces and divides, thus generating the rest of the epithelium. But if the cells grow in an uncontrolled fashion, they might form a tumor.

To balance this yin-yang, cells have a complex set of mechanisms that determine how quickly they grow and reproduce. Some cellular genes promote cell growth and cycling; others suppress it. When an outside factor—like a mutation on the controlling gene—causes expression of too much or too many of the growth-promoting genes, a tumor may form. (We sometimes call these genes *oncogenes*, since the prefix *onco* means "cancer.")

On the other hand, if you have inadequate levels of the

growth-suppressing genes, you may also get too much cell cycling. (We sometimes call these genes *tumor suppressors.*) This could happen if these genes mutate, functionally knocking them out, or if they disappear from your genome altogether. Mutations could also affect the DNA that determines the level of tumor suppressors, leading to levels that are too low. The p53 and pRB genes are both examples of tumor suppressor genes, since they both act to slow down cell cycling and cell division.

How does HPV interact with p53 and pRB to cause tumors? This is an extraordinarily complex topic, and hundreds of research papers have covered the subject. I'll try to present a greatly simplified version of how these interactions may play out in real life, and this is shown in figure 1.7.

Suppose that after you finish your course in HPV 101, you decide to take a break and catch a few rays. You go out into the bright sunshine and hang out for a few hours. Let's say that you didn't put on any sunscreen. The sun is constantly bathing your face with its ultraviolet (UV) radiation, which can damage the DNA of your facial skin. Rarely, the UV irradiation causes enough mutations—in one or more of the cellular genes that control cell cycling and division—that the damage may eventually lead to cancer. So why don't we all get cancer?

Part of the reason comes back to p53. When UV irradiation damages the facial skin's basal cell DNA, the cells respond to this challenge by functionally saying to themselves, "Whoa! We've been hurt. Let's stop dividing until our DNA is fixed. I mean, if we continue to divide, our bad DNA will be passed on to our daughter or son cells. If we

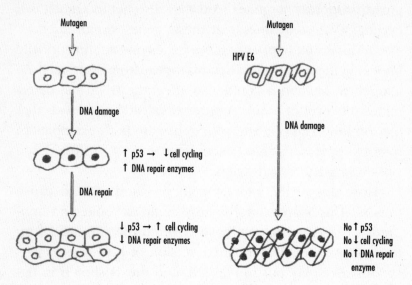

Figure 1.7: How the HPV E6 Protein May Contribute to Cancer.
Our epithelium is constantly exposed to DNA-damaging events, and the
DNA damage may contribute to the development of cancer. Shown on
the left of the diagram is how cells react to DNA damage to repair
themselves. When the DNA of the cells is damaged, the level of the p53
protein in the cell rises. Nuclei with damaged DNA are shown as
darker than nuclei with normal DNA. The p53 protein stops the cells
from dividing and increases the level of DNA repair proteins. Once the
DNA is repaired, p53 levels in the cell return to normal. The cell nuclei
are shown as lighter in color again and the now-repaired cell is free to
continue dividing. On the right of the diagram are cells infected with
HPV that are producing the HPV E6 protein, depicted by hatched lines
in the cytoplasm surrounding the cell nucleus. Since expression of the
HPV E6 protein leads to the destruction of p53, there is no p53 in these
cells to protect them. If there is DNA damage in these cells (again
shown as dark nuclei) the cells continue to divide without repairing
their DNA (the nuclei remain dark), propagating the DNA damage.
Eventually some of this damage might lead to the development of
cancer. (Illustration by Ira C. Smith.)

continue to have more DNA-damaging events, damage to our DNA will accumulate, we might damage our cell control mechanisms, and then—well, we might spin out of control and become cancerous. I don't think we oughta let that happen."

Think of it this way: If you're not feeling well, your doctor will probably tell you that bed rest is the best medicine. Stay off your feet, sleep, and your body will be able to focus on getting you well rather than generating enough energy to get you well *and* to get you through a rough day at work. If you just keep going, never take medicine or rest even a little, you'll probably get sicker and your illness will last longer.

So how do the cells respond to DNA damage? Typically, the cell senses DNA damage and responds by increasing its p53 levels. First, p53 stops the cell from dividing, and second, p53 turns on other cellular genes that specialize in repairing the damaged DNA. Once the damage is repaired, p53 levels drop and the cells are free to continue dividing as good as new.

So how does HPV fit into this? The E6 protein of HPV not only attaches to and inactivates the p53 protein, but also leads to its physical destruction. In essence, when E6 attaches to p53, it also attaches a molecular signal to p53 that tells the cell to destroy it—in other words, E6 literally gives p53 the kiss of death! Now imagine that an HPV-infected cell containing that E6 protein undergoes DNA damage. Since E6 is present, no p53 is available to help repair the cell as described above. Instead, the cell continues dividing inappropriately, and the DNA damage passes on to succeeding generations of cells.

Like the effect of E6 on p53, the HPV E7 protein inactivates the pRB protein. Like p53, pRB helps suppress cell cycling and division. However, E7 does not lead to the destruction of pRB—just its inactivation. Like the effect of E6 on p53, the binding of E7 to pRB also leads to inappropriate cell division in the face of cellular DNA damage. So, in effect, the HPV E6 and E7 proteins provide a kind of one-two punch to normal cellular growth control mechanisms. In other words, with oncogenic HPV types, the cell "doctor" that tells your cell to rest has been held hostage by HPV genes. So your cells continue on their way, allowing their nuclei to produce more damaged DNA and producing more mutated cells.

Ultimately, the resulting cellular DNA damage may lead to the development of cervical cancer. Therefore, the HPV E6 and E7 proteins probably contribute to the development of cancer in an indirect manner through inducing "genomic instability," and that's what directly leads to cancer development.

I mentioned sunbathing the skin of your face. Clearly the cervix doesn't get exposed to sun. But does the cervix get exposed to DNA-damaging elements? Probably. One such example is smoking. Remember how I said that smoking is a risk factor for dysplasia and cancer? Get this: When a woman smokes a cigarette, her levels of tar and nicotine in the cervical mucus may be *as high or higher* than levels of tar and nicotine in her bloodstream! In other words, potential tobacco-related, DNA-damaging carcinogens are bathing the cervix exactly where you *least* want them—in the presence of cells infected with HPV, that are expressing the HPV E6 protein, and which consequently have no p53 to protect them.

Interestingly, this also helps to explain why some HPV types, such as HPV 16 and 18, can cause cancer and why others, such as HPV 6 and 11, do not. Again, this is an over-simplification, but it turns out that the E6 and E7 proteins of the cancer-causing HPV types are much more efficient at inactivating p53 and pRB than the E6 and E7 proteins of the nononcogenic, low-risk HPV types.

All of this is happening on a cellular level, so the infection is considered to be subclinical—without any outward manifestation of symptoms. In women, the infection is in your cervix, so you can't see it there; in men, it's barely visible on the penis. A subclinical infection is particularly insidious, since it can occur and progress without a person ever knowing he or she has it.

Transmission of HPV: "When Am I Infectious?"

As I said earlier, the most infectious stage is probably when you have a wart or mild dysplasia. Moderate and severe dysplasia produce infectious virus as well, but not as much as mild dysplasia.

You're probably wondering, "Am I infectious if I have HPV infection but no signs of any disease?" We don't really know. Most HPVologists are inclined to say "possibly," but clearly at a much lower level than if you have dysplasia. Theoretically, little or no mature virus particle forms in normal skin, so if that skin contains HPV, only naked HPV

DNA will be shed from it. While naked DNA could be taken up by your partner's genital skin cells and cause an infection, this is probably much less common than infections caused by mature HPV particles. The problem is, we don't really *know* when HPV becomes contagious. Consequently, we don't know when it *stops* being contagious.

The only way to scientifically test for HPV transmission is to find women with known active HPV infection, send them out into the world to have sex with virginal men, and test each of those men to see if they acquired HPV. The experiment could also be done the other way around. Scientifically, that methodology is not 100 percent accurate. Morally and ethically, it's out of the question.

A major concern of my patients is, understandably, how long they'll be infectious. Can they spread HPV for the rest of their lives, anytime? Unfortunately, I can't give a straight yes or no answer to that. I can only say . . . *maybe.*

Many doctors take the position that HPV is most contagious in the months after you acquire your own HPV infection and develop dysplasia. Once you've had three or four normal Pap smears in a row, you're probably no longer infectious. However, since you may still have HPV even if you have a normal Pap smear, there's still a very small possibility that you could transmit HPV to a partner.

If you're having regular sex with someone, it's very likely that they'll get HPV. In a monogamous, long-term relationship like marriage, that's usually not a major issue, since both you and your partner know that, with due vigilance, HPV rarely leads to anything more harmful than an abnormal Pap smear.

Once you have been diagnosed with HPV, my advice is

to assume that you will always be infectious. This, of course, means you'll have to discuss HPV with a potential sexual partner, which always leads to . . .

The Condom Question

The condom question is a double-edged sword when it comes to HPV. Unlike the human immunodeficiency virus, HIV, which is spread through bodily fluids such as semen and blood, HPV is spread by surface contact, basically skin-to-skin contact. The problem with a condom, of course, is that a man can have a subclinical lesion at the base of his penis or on his scrotum, beyond the reach of the condom. If that skin comes in contact with a woman's vulva or vagina, then skin-to-skin contact has occurred, and transmission can happen despite condom use.

Condoms probably do help to reduce the risk of HPV transmission, but clearly they don't do a good enough job by themselves.

No, condoms are *not* a foolproof method of protection against HPV infection. That said, barring abstinence, latex condoms are the single most effective protection against STDs—HPV included—currently available.

Which leaves you, of course, in a difficult spot, especially if you're young, single, and sexually active (which, incidentally, is the group with the highest HPV infection rate). My best advice is this: Talk to your partner before having sex. The discussion can be extremely difficult, especially at first, but think of it this way: Wouldn't you rather know if your partner has signs of HPV infection such as warts or dysplasia, or had them in the past? One of the problems with this advice, as I'll discuss later in the book, is that many men have HPV infection but don't know it. So your partner may be answering perfectly honestly that he is not aware of having HPV infection, but he could still be harboring an infectious lesion on his penis or scrotum.

As for the condom issue, ask yourself this: Would you jump without a parachute on the off chance that it might not open on the way down? Of course not. Be smart and be safe.

As I said, if one partner in a monogamous relationship has HPV, it is probable that both of them will have it eventually, so the decision to use condoms is entirely up to them.

Risk Factors for Acquiring HPV

Of course, some practices put you more at risk for getting HPV infection than others. After all, in the days when nuns entered the convent as young girls, they rarely got cervical cancer, and that's simply because they abstained from sex. Keep in mind, too, that the risk factors for developing dysplasia (and/or cancer) and acquiring HPV overlap, but are not the same. Think of it this way: Because HPV is a risk factor for dysplasia, all of the risk factors for HPV are also risks for dysplasia. But not all the risk factors for dysplasia are factors for HPV.

Although HPV is necessary for dysplasia to develop, it's not the only factor. In medicalese, we say that HPV infection is "necessary but insufficient." That's really good news because most sexually active women get HPV infection, but only a small percentage of women will develop dysplasia, and an even smaller proportion will develop cervical cancer (see fig. 1.4). Imagine the medical disaster if all women who got HPV developed cervical cancer!

There are several risk factors for acquiring HPV, and almost all of them involve sexual contact.

What Is Sex?

Seems like a dumb question, doesn't it? But in reality, the answer is complicated—and terribly important. Because "sex" means different things to different people. Some people equate sex with having vaginal intercourse. Others define it as any kind of intimate physical contact between two people. From the HPV standpoint, the definition of sex is quite liberal. Since I already said HPV spreads by skin-to-skin contact, many forms of sexual contact could lead to acquisition of HPV. This could include genital rubbing (frottage) with or without vaginal intercourse. This means that any kind of sexual activity could lead to transmission of HPV—man to woman, woman to man, woman to woman, and man to man.

Can you get HPV by being touched by someone with their finger or with a sexual toy? Remember, you won't get one of the HPV types that lives on someone's hand in your genital region, because HPV types usually prefer their own body part. But it *is* possible that hands could spread genital HPV types if someone touches their own infected genital skin and then touches the genital skin of their uninfected partner. In this context, the hand is serving as a "carrier" for the genital HPV types. We don't really know how often this happens, but it's probably uncommon. Likewise, it's possible that in *rare* circumstances, towels could spread HPV if a person vigorously dries himself or herself off and then *immediately* towels off his or her partner. But I want to stress that these modes of transmission are probably quite rare. Doctors suspect that genital HPV types don't live for very long by themselves outside of a person's anogenital region. For example, we know that HPV can't be acquired from a toilet seat.

Modes of Acquiring HPV Infection

You'll *most likely* get HPV from . . .

- Giving or receiving unprotected vaginal intercourse
- Giving or receiving unprotected anal intercourse
- Perinatal (mother-to-child) transmission
- Another area of your own genitals (spread from an infected area to an uninfected area through shaving, scratching, or other methods)

You *may* get HPV from . . .

- Fingers or other uninfected body parts
- Giving or receiving protected vaginal intercourse
- Giving or receiving protected anal intercourse
- Giving or receiving oral sex
- Rubbing genitals
- Sex toys

You may *rarely* get HPV from . . .

- Sharing towels

You'll *never* get HPV from . . .

- A toilet seat
- A public telephone
- A toad or other animal

When in doubt, ask your doctor!

Autoinfection is another way to get HPV infection. That's medicalese for "infecting yourself" by spreading infection from one area of your body to another area of your own body. If you're infected in one part of your genitals with an HPV type, you can spread it yourself to other parts of your genitals. For example, shaving can possibly spread HPV. If you shave your pubic hair, and you touch an infected area with the razor, you could spread it if you knick yourself with it somewhere else in the genital region. Likewise, you could spread HPV infection from the cervix to the anal canal or vice versa, through wiping or natural movement of fluids. If you're a man, you could spread HPV infection from your penis to your anus or vice versa by scratching yourself in a shedding, infected area, and then scratching an uninfected area. Women can, of course, also infect themselves by scratching.

What about oral sex? Oral sex can spread HPV from the genital region to the mouth, where it can lead to oral warts, oral dysplasia or even oral cancer, but again, not very often. Conversely, oral sex with someone who has oral HPV infection can lead to transmission to the genital region.

Risk Factors for Acquiring HPV Infection

- **Multiple partners.** The plain truth is this: The more partners you have, the higher chance you have of getting HPV. It's a simple matter of increasing the odds.
- **Sexual contact with a partner who's had multiple partners.** Remember the saying "Every time you have sex with someone, you're having sex with everyone they've had sex with." I'd amend that statement to read "sexual contact," rather than "sex."
- **Younger age at first intercourse.** Women who begin to have sex at a younger age, such as during the teen years, are at increased risk of acquiring HPV infection. The cervix in younger women is biologically immature and its cervical transformation zone is bigger, more exposed, and therefore more vulnerable. Also, younger women who have not yet been exposed to HPV may not have any natural immunity to the virus in the form of antibodies.
- **Unprotected sexual contact.** Although condoms are not infallible, especially with a skin-contact virus like HPV, condoms are the best protection you have against most STDs. *Use them.*
- **Sexual contact with an infected partner.** Communication between partners can go a long way toward reducing your risk. For instance, if he's *your* first and only partner, but he's had intercourse with multiple women, then your risk increases. If one of his partners had cervical cancer, or if he has had penile warts or cancer, then it's likely he has HPV. Bottom line: The "contagion factor" of HPV is still unknown. If there's a chance that you or your partner has ever been diagnosed with HPV, you'll have to entertain the idea that the virus could be lying dormant and is still contagious. Although discussing this with your partner is the best approach to taking appropriate precautions, you'd be wise to simply assume your partner has HPV infection.

I'm sure these risk factors sound familiar. They're virtually the same as every other STD out there. Let's face it: Knowing your partner, having fewer partners, and using condoms are the best routes to avoiding STDs. Be smart and be safe.

What about risk factors for dysplasia? As I said earlier, HPV infection is necessary but insufficient for development of dysplasia. Although risk factors for HPV and dysplasia largely overlap, a few other factors also increase the risk of developing dysplasia among women with HPV infection, including smoking, use of birth control pills (a relatively small increase in risk), and immunosuppression (a weakened immune system).

Risk Factors for Developing Dysplasia

- **HPV infection.** If you have HPV, you have the one factor that is *necessary* for dysplasia, and therefore cancer, to develop. However, other factors are important, too.
- **History of STDs.** STDs, particularly with an organism called chlamydia trachomatis, can weaken the cervix and make it vulnerable to HPV-induced cellular changes. Although your current history cannot be changed, more communication with your sexual partners and using condoms can prevent future STDs.
- **Smoking.** Smoking weakens your immune system. It fills your body with carcinogens and accelerates the degeneration of normal cells into abnormal cells. Smoking contributes to the development of cancer, whether it's cervical, lung, oral, or otherwise. *Smoking kills.*
- **Stress.** Psychological stress may weaken your immune system. Do what you can to lower the stress level in your life.
- **Family history.** If your family has a history of cervical cancer, your chances of developing dysplasia (and thus cancer) may be increased. Lucky for you, though, you know what the risk factors are and can stop the development early on.

- **Poor nutrition and/or obesity.** Some studies have shown that a balanced diet that includes lots of fruits and vegetables, folic acid, and vitamins A, C, and E can increase your cervix's ability to fight off the HPV infection. Mom was right—eat your fruits and vegetables!
- **Oral contraceptive use.** The relationship between birth control pills and cervical cancer has been heavily debated. One reason that oral contraceptive use is a risk factor could be that fewer women who use oral contraceptives use condoms, thus increasing their chances of transmitting HPV. Another reason is that the steroids in the pill may stimulate production of HPV proteins. In either case, the effect is likely to be real, but weak.
- **Age.** Although more young women have HPV, cervical cancer and moderate or severe dysplasia are far more common in women thirty years or older. Loss of immunity and menopause could contribute to this increased incidence, so older women are especially reminded to get Pap smears.
- **HIV, pregnancy, and other immunity-compromised conditions.** As with the poor nutrition, decreased immunity means increased risk. Many HIV-positive patients, pregnant women, and recent recipients of organ transplants experience dysplasia because their immune systems aren't as capable of keeping HPV in check.
- **Low socioeconomic status.** Although poor general health contributes to a decrease in immunity, poor *health care*—meaning the lack of insurance, money, and regular doctor visits—increases your risk of advancing beyond dysplasia to cervical cancer. Women with less money and access to health care are less likely to get Paps and are therefore less likely to find potentially treatable dysplasia and cancer in its early stages. In developing countries, cervical cancer is one of the most common killers of women simply because they don't have the means to get regular Paps.

When Do Women Get Cervical HPV Infection, Dysplasia, and Cervical Cancer?

What follows is a summary of some of the information I've already given you (also shown in fig. 1.4). First, let's look at HPV infection over time. Basically, most sexually active women acquire HPV infection at some point in their lives. In fact, most women acquire the infection from one or more of their first few sexual partners. It's not surprising, then, that the women with the highest proportion of HPV infection are those under the age of twenty-four years.

But if you look at women over the age of thirty years, you'll notice that the proportion of women who have HPV infection drops off steadily over time. Why? They've probably developed an immune response to HPV and have either cleared the virus from their body or are at least keeping the virus to levels that make it undetectable by currently available tests.

What's not seen in the diagram in figure 1.4 is recent evidence that some women over the age of sixty begin to have detectable HPV again. It's not clear why, but it could be a loss of immune response to HPV due to the effects of aging. Or, it's possible that they may have been exposed to a new HPV type—sex certainly doesn't stop after the age of thirty! Overall, though, most women have their HPV infection when they're in their teens and early twenties. It's the women who continue to have HPV infection after the age of thirty who worry us the most. These are the women at highest risk of developing severe dysplasia and cancer.

Now let's look at the relationship between dysplasia and age, shown in the second and third lines from the top in figure 1.4. The proportion of women who have detectable dysplasia at some point in their lives is much smaller than the proportion of women who acquire HPV. In other words, many women may have HPV, but fewer develop a negative reaction to it.

Why is this the case? It probably comes back to the immune system—most mild dysplasia (also termed CIN 1 or low-grade squamous intraepithelial lesions [LSIL]) develops early on after acquiring HPV infection. HPV proteins are made in these lesions, and the immune system kicks in to destroy the cells making the HPV proteins. So the lesions develop and then go away—at least most of them do—and most of these low-grade lesions resolve by themselves by the time a woman reaches the age of thirty. The same is true for moderate and severe dysplasia (CIN 2 and 3, or high-grade squamous intraepithelial lesions [HSIL]), except that they tend to peak later in life than the low-grade lesions and they don't spontaneously regress as often. Fortunately, high-grade lesions such as moderate and severe dysplasia are more rare than low-grade lesions, and much rarer than HPV infection itself.

Now let's look at the relationship between cancer and age, shown in the bottom line. Here you'll notice that cervical cancer tends to peak even later in life than HPV infection and dysplasia. Thank goodness it's also much rarer than dysplasia. Nevertheless, as I mentioned earlier, rare as it is, cervical cancer does kill about five thousand women every year in the United States, and many more in developing countries.

Since there's a great deal of HPV infection and relatively little severe dysplasia among women in their late teens and early twenties, much of the cervical cancer control efforts are focused on women who are thirty and older, who continue to have HPV infection, and who especially continue to have dysplasia. Women older than the age of sixty are also carefully followed since, as I said, a second peak of HPV infection and dysplasia is being noticed in this age group.

Conclusion

In this one chapter, you've learned more about HPV and how it works than many doctors know. Why bother giving you all this information about virology and cell differentiation and DNA? Because, as I said before, knowing what's happening in your body gives you a more solid sense of control. After reading this chapter, you won't be frightened or intimidated by your doctor's report, nor will you feel confused when he or she says you have dysplasia. You'll know almost *exactly* what's happening in your body, right down to the nuclei in your cells.

A quick analogy: It's two in the morning. You hear someone climb into your living room window and begin rifling through your valuables. You call the police, hide under your bed, and they take away the burglar. Would you rather the police officers say, "OK, we got him," or "We got him, and here's a list of the things he stole, and these are the rooms he went through, and this is what he looks like"? Personally, I like to know what's going on in my home.

So why shouldn't you afford your body the same respect?

Questions to Ask Your Doctor

- Am I at risk for getting HPV?
- What should I tell my partner?
- What are the safest sexual practices to prevent HPV transmission?
- If I get a new partner and we use condoms, will he still get HPV?
- When is HPV infection considered "latent," and what does latent infection mean for me?
- Will I have HPV for the rest of my life?

CHAPTER TWO

Pap Smears 101

As is the case with most tests doctors perform, I'd wager that many women aren't even sure what happens during a Pap smear, even though they've been having them for ten or twenty years. Ignorance only contributes to fear and discomfort—kind of like your five-year-old not knowing what's in the closet. As long as you show your child that the only thing in the closet is clothes and some shoes, he won't be frightened—or at least he'll be less frightened. But as long as the door's closed and the light's out, his imagination can run wild with scenarios.

More knowledge leads to less fear—and since you'll have the power to ask educated questions, more knowledge also leads to better health.

First Things First: Your Cervix

Your cervix (shown in fig. 2.1), a relatively small area sandwiched between the vagina and the uterus, is actually the lowest portion of the uterus—kind of a hallway to your vagina, allowing menstrual blood to flow out of the uterus. (*Cervix* actually means "neck.") The cervix's top layer is the epithelium I described in chapter 1.

What Does Your Cervix Do for You?

As the gateway to the uterus, the cervix has several functions. With the help of cervical mucus, it protects the uterus from infections. During pregnancy, the cervix serves the vital function of helping to hold in the fetus. When the cervix becomes too lax (as a result of some of the treatments that will be discussed later in this book), this is known as *cervical incompetence*, and the baby may be delivered prematurely. If the cervix becomes scarred (also as a result of some of the treatments that will be discussed later in this book), it may block menstrual flow.

The cervix has two different kinds of epithelium: columnar and squamous. The columnar cells have a tall, thin appearance that resembles a column. These cells line a part of the cervix known as the *endocervical canal*, a tubelike structure leading from the outer part of the cervix (*exocervix*) to the uterus (see fig. 1.5).

The endocervical columnar cells, like glandular cells, primarily produce cervical mucus. Among other things, cervical mucus protects your cervix against bacteria and sexu-

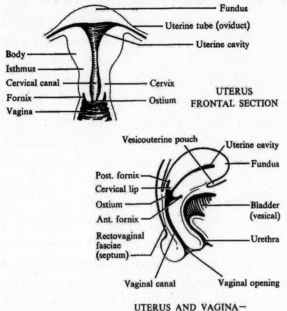

Figure 2.1: Female Reproductive Organs. *The upper panel shows upper vagina, cervix, and uterus. The lower panel shows a side view of the cervix leading to the uterus. (Reprinted by permission of the McGraw-Hill Companies. This illustration was previously printed in Pansky, Ben,* Review of Gross Anatomy, *1979.)*

ally transmitted pathogens. (Because it acts like a gland, the columnar epithelium is sometimes referred to as *glandular epithelium,* a term we'll see later when we cover types of abnormal Pap smears.)

The outer part of the cervix, or exocervix, is covered by squamous epithelium, the multilayered epithelium described in chapter 1. As I said earlier, the transformation zone (TZ) occurs where the columnar epithelium meets the squamous epithelium.

During the course of a woman's life, the relationship between the columnar and squamous epithelium changes, as does the TZ. Before puberty, the columnar epithelium extends beyond the endocervical canal and onto the exocervix. When your body prepares itself for sexual activity during puberty, one cell layer isn't enough to properly protect your cervix. In the transformation zone, the thicker, more adaptive multilayered squamous epithelium replaces the columnar epithelium, and two layers form: the columnar epithelium at the bottom layer, and the squamous epithelium on the top layer.

This transformation results in the development of squamous tissue, which gradually reaches maturity through a woman's late adolescence. During puberty, the TZ is especially large and exposed. This may be one reason why adolescent girls are at such high risk of acquiring sexually transmitted infections, including HPV.

As a woman matures biologically, the TZ continues to change, and in many cases, gets smaller. As it does, some or all of it may retract into the endocervical canal. At that point, your doctor may have trouble seeing it during a Pap smear, and as you know, the TZ is one of the prime areas for HPV infection. If your doctor cannot properly assess this area, he or she may need to use special diagnostic techniques to rule out the presence of dysplasia, described in chapter 5.

Like the squamous epithelium, the columnar epithelium can also be infected with HPV, resulting in a different form of dysplasia or even cancer known as *adenocarcinoma* of the cervix (cancer of the mucus-producing columnar cells). Interestingly, the spectrum of HPV types associated with adenocarcinoma is a little different from those of squamous cell carcinoma. For example, infection with HPV 18 is found more often in adenocarcinoma than it is in squamous cell carcinoma. Because of the potential to develop cervical cancer arising in the endocervical canal, the endocervical canal is assessed as part of the routine Pap smear, described below.

Prevention of Cervical Cancer: How and Why

Now you know that sexual activity leads to a high risk of HPV infection, and you know that in most women HPV infection doesn't lead to serious problems . . . but for some, HPV leads to dysplasia.

Most women who develop mild dysplasia spontaneously regress: The lesion goes away by itself. Some will progress to moderate or severe dysplasia, however, and some women may skip over mild or moderate dysplasia all together; they go directly to severe. And some undiagnosed or untreated moderate or severe dysplasia—especially severe—will progress to invasive cervical cancer.

Your goal—and your doctor's—is to prevent cervical cancer. Mild dysplasia doesn't progress directly to invasive cancer, but moderate or severe dysplasia can, and efforts to prevent cervical cancer focus on identifying and treating moderate or severe cases before they can progress further.

That's where the Pap smear comes in. Remember that the other term for cervical Pap smear is *cervical cytology*. The test allows the cytologist or cytopathologist to look for signs of abnormalities in the cervical cells, particularly changes consistent with HSIL. Why is it so useful? The answer's simple—because it's quick, inexpensive, and relatively easy to perform. (I say "relatively" because the Pap smear does have some problems, which I'll discuss later.)

What *Is* a Pap Smear?

Most women probably don't think much about their cervices outside of their yearly Pap smears. Why would they? But before George Papanicolaou invented the Pap smear, or cervical cytology, in the 1940s, cervical cancer was the *number one* killer of women in the world. Since the Pap smear, the rate of death from cervical cancer has dropped by 75 percent in the United States, but worldwide, it's the second most common cancer in women, and the most common cancer in some developing countries. Worldwide, 452,000 new cases and more than 234,000 deaths occur each year, and 80 percent of these cases are found in developing countries that don't have the means for regular screening (Miller 2000).

With the resources we have in the United States, we have the means to get a Pap smear every year. Bottom line? Regular Pap smears save lives.

What Happens during a Pap Smear?

At this point, I'm going to switch terminology on you, and hope that you don't get too confused. Remember that we

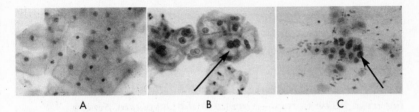

A   B   C

Figure 2.2: Normal Cervical Cells, Mild Dysplasia, and Severe Dysplasia in Cervical Pap Smears. *Figure 2.2A shows a Pap smear that is normal. It contains many epithelial cells that have a normal size and a normal nucleus and no sign of changes induced by HPV. Figure 2.2B shows a Pap smear containing mild dysplasia. Shown with an arrow is a koilocyte that is typical of mild dysplasia. The cell has an enlarged irregular nucleus surrounded by a halo. Figure 2.2C shows a Pap smear containing severe dysplasia. Shown with an arrow is a small cell that contains an enlarged nucleus, typical of severe dysplasia. (Photos courtesy of Dr. Teresa Darragh, University of California, San Francisco.)*

use the Bethesda terminology to grade Pap smears, as opposed to the terminology we use for biopsy tissues. In other words, for Pap smears we use the terms *LSIL* and *HSIL* instead of *mild, moderate,* or *severe,* the words that are used to classify dysplasia.

In as few words as possible: During a Pap smear, a doctor scrapes the surface cells of the exocervix, endocervix, and TZ and puts them on a slide for examination by the cytotechnologist and cytopathologist. The sample is essentially random and the cells are placed at random on the slide. The cytotechnologist and/or cytopathologist looks at the cells on the slide to look for signs of LSIL and especially HSIL. (A series of Pap smears showing different results ranging from normal to HSIL is shown in fig. 2.2.)

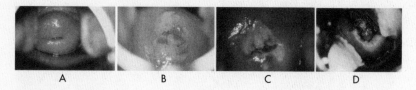

Figure 2.3: The Cervix—Normal, Mild Dysplasia, Severe Dysplasia, and Invasive Cancer as Seen through the Colposcope. A vaginal speculum is inserted and the cervix is examined through the colposcope under magnification, after application of 5 percent acetic acid (vinegar). Seen in figure 2.3B is a cervix with mild dysplasia. Figure 2.3C shows a cervix with severe dysplasia. Figure 2.3D shows an invasive cancer with underlying tissue destruction due to invasion by the cancerous cells. (Photos 2.3A, 2.3B, 2.3C courtesy of Dr. Teresa Darragh, University of California, San Francisco. Photo 2.3D reprinted by permission of Mosby-Year Books, Inc., St. Louis, Missouri, 64146. Photo originally appeared in DiSaia and Creasman, Clinical Gynecologic Oncology, *Fifth edition, 1997.*)

What Happens If Your Pap Smear Comes Back Abnormal?

I'll discuss this in great detail later in the book. But basically, many women with abnormal Pap smears will have a follow-up test known as a *colposcopy*. As you know, a Pap smear is a bunch of cells smeared on a slide. The cytotechnologist or cytopathologist can determine if there are abnormal cells on the slide, but they can't tell where in the cervix or vagina they came from. So the next step is to perform the colposcopy, in which the doctor directly examines the cervix and vagina under magnification. If your doctor sees the source of those abnormal cells, he or she may take a sample of the tissue, known as a *biopsy*. The results of this biopsy usually determine what, if any, treatment you'll require. Again, all of this is covered in greater detail later in

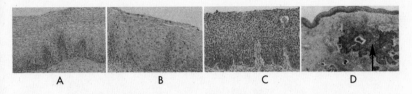

A   B   C   D

Figure 2.4: Biopsies Showing Normal Tissue, Mild Dysplasia, Severe Dysplasia, and Cancer of the Cervix. *Figure 2.4A shows a normal cervical biopsy. The epithelial cells look healthy and show normal maturation. In figure 2.4B the biopsy shows mild dysplasia with koilocytes and relatively normal cellular maturation. In figure 2.4C, the biopsy shows severe dysplasia with replacement of the epithelium with small cells with an enlarged nucleus, and lack of normal cell maturation in the surface layers. Fig 2.4D shows an invasive cancer. Note the patch of epithelial cells underneath the basement membrane shown by the arrow that have invaded the tissues underlying the epithelium. These cells may continue to divide and spread if the cancer is not treated. (Photos 2.4A, 2.4B, 2.4C courtesy of Dr. Teresa Darragh, University of California, San Francisco. Photo 2.4D reprinted by permission of Mosby-Year Books, Inc., St. Louis, Missouri, 64146. Photo originally appeared in DiSaia and Creasman,* Clinical Gynecologic Oncology, *Fifth edition, 1997.)*

the book. The appearance of the normal cervix and examples of cervices that show mild dysplasia, severe dysplasia, and cancer as seen through the colposcope are shown in figure 2.3.

Once the lesion is identified, your doctor obtains a tissue sample of the lesion (a biopsy) and, based on the results of the tissue examination, creates a treatment plan. Figure 2.4 shows a series of cervical biopsies, ranging from normal to mild dysplasia to severe dysplasia to cancer. Treatment decisions are almost always based on the results of the biopsy, not on the Pap smear. The role of the Pap smear, then, essentially is to determine if a woman requires colposcopy.

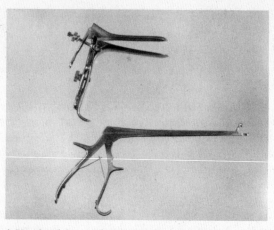

Figure 2.5: A Vaginal Speculum and Biopsy Forceps. *On the upper part of this picture is a typical cervical speculum that is inserted to allow clinicians to see the cervix to obtain a cervical Pap smear. On the bottom part of the picture is an instrument used to obtain biopsies (pieces of cervical tissue) for examination by the pathologist under a microscope. (Author's photo.)*

That's the short answer. Now for the long answer . . .

What most women believe is a Pap smear is actually a combination of a Pap smear and a Pap *test*. The smear is the actual sample from your vagina and cervix; the test is the examination of that sample.

During your yearly checkup with your doctor, you'll receive a pelvic examination—a full investigation of your reproductive health—and this includes the Pap smear. (Although we are using the term *doctor* here, many health professionals can perform Pap smears, including nurse practitioners and physician's assistants. After you lie back on the table and put your feet in the stirrups, your doctor will insert a *speculum* to hold open the walls of your vagina. The

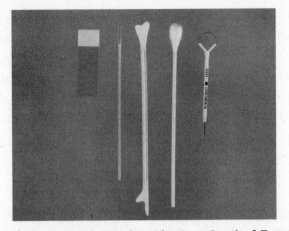

Figure 2.6: Instruments Used to Obtain a Cervical Pap Smear and to Treat Cervical Disease with the Loop Electrosurgical Excision Procedure (LEEP). Shown left to right in this figure are instruments used to collect cervical cells for a Pap smear—a glass slide, a cervical cytobrush, and a spatula. These are used to scrape cells off the surface of the cervix. The cells are placed on a glass slide or in a bottle of cell preservative. To the right of the spatula is a cotton swab used to remove mucus from the cervix and on the far right is an electrical wire used in the loop electrosurgical excision procedure (LEEP) to remove cervical dysplasia. (Author's photo.)

speculum is shown in figure 2.5. The speculum may cause some discomfort, but your doctor will warm or lubricate it to make insertion a little more comfortable for you.

Using a brush, spatula, or long cotton swab to brush against your cervix, your doctor will obtain cervical cells and smear them on a slide. These are shown in figure 2.6. At that point, they preserve the cells by either immersing the slide in alcohol or spraying the slide with a fixative (sometimes hairspray!), and then send it to lab. There, a cytotechnologist (a technician specializing in identifying cell abnormalities) will study the slide, systematically inspecting the entire smear for any abnormal cells. Abnormal smears, as well as a random sampling of normal smears, are then reexamined by a cytopathologist (a doctor specializing in the interpretation of abnormal cells on a slide). They report the results to your doctor. The entire process takes about five days. *Your* involvement takes about five minutes. Pap smears can be uncomfortable, but they're worth it.

How Are Pap Smears Interpreted? The Bethesda System

Without basic information on the most current classification system of Pap smears, you'll have a tough time following the rest of the book. So it'll probably be useful to refer back to the chart on page 28 showing the Pap smear and biopsy classification systems. Once you know the Bethesda system, you'll even understand your own Pap smear report.

The "class" system simply rated the cell changes on a scale of one to five. Now we use the "Bethesda" system, a detailed system for naming each stage of cellular change. Instead of saying "negative," for instance, and labeling a Pap smear normal, the Bethesda system has two categories for smears that have no signs of SIL. One category recognizes perfectly healthy cells with no changes, and these are called "normal." Another category recognizes cellular changes usually associated with cervical infection (other than HPV), atrophy (usually during the low-estrogen state of menopause), and repair, but which are benign.

It's also important to distinguish between a Pap smear

and an HPV test: An HPV test, discussed later in this book, looks directly for HPV DNA or RNA. The Pap test looks for changes in the cells that have been caused by HPV, but it doesn't look for HPV itself.

> A Pap test does *not* look for HPV per se, but looks for changes in the epithelial cells induced by HPV.

The following chapters will describe the different stages of a Pap smear: unsatisfactory, normal, abnormal, all the way through to cervical cancer. Some stages warrant more discussion than others do, but every classification of your Pap smear is distinct and important. Keep in mind that if your Pap is in a category *not* linked to HPV (such as normal or unsatisfactory), that doesn't necessarily mean that you don't have HPV, or that you're not at risk for developing an abnormal Pap smear at a later point.

How Often Should I Have a Pap Smear?

The American College of Obstetrics and Gynecology and the American Cancer Society both recommend that all women begin yearly Pap tests at age eighteen or when they become sexually active, whichever occurs earlier. If a woman has had three negative annual Pap tests in a row, the test may be done less often, at the judgment of a woman's health care provider. Here's where having an open line of communication with your provider will be critical: He or she will need to know as much as possible about your risk factors for HPV infection to make the best recommendation for your Pap smear screening interval.

Women who've had hysterectomies may also benefit from Pap smears. Even though the cervix has been removed, a Pap test can examine cells shed from the vagina for signs of HPV-induced changes.

Some data suggest that women who have sex with women (WSW) are at risk of HPV-associated genital disease. WSW can transmit HPV to each other, and they're also at risk if they've previously had or continue to have one or more male sexual partners. Some doctors believe that WSW aren't at risk of cervical disease since they assume that they don't have male sexual partners, but that's not always the case. Regardless of whether a woman has had male partners or not, WSW are at risk of HPV infection, they do need Pap smears, and all of the information in this book that applies to women who have sex with men also applies to WSW.

HIV-positive women are advised to have a comprehensive gynecologic examination and a Pap smear as part of their initial medical evaluation. If initial results are normal, at least one additional Pap should be obtained six months later to exclude a false-negative result on the initial smear. If the second smear is normal, HIV-infected women could have annual smears, similar to HIV-negative women. If the initial or follow-up cytology shows ASCUS or SIL, the woman should be referred for a colposcopy.

How Accurate Is My Pap Smear?

In the last few years, you may have read horror stories about women who had a "normal" Pap test and then less than a year later were diagnosed with invasive cervical cancer. Clearly something went wrong with the system. As with any clinical test, each step in the test process has its own set of problems, which I'll tell you about in a moment. Basically the Pap is not 100 percent accurate on an individual basis, but over time, its statistical sensitivity increases. Here's what I mean:

Suppose that each Pap test is only 60 percent sensitive (a low figure, but not that uncommon in many institutions). That means that for every one hundred women with dysplasia, sixty will be told that they have an abnormal Pap smear, and they may be referred for colposcopy for further investigation. The remaining forty women will be told that they have a normal Pap smear and, presumably, will not have any further investigation done until their next routine Pap smear. These women have what is called a *false-negative* Pap smear. This means that those forty women will have dysplasia but will go untreated.

Obviously, this is not a good thing.

Suppose that these women have their Pap smear repeated twelve months later. If the Pap smear is only 60 percent sensitive, then the chance that an individual woman will have two false-negative Pap smears in a row is $0.6 \times 0.6 = .36$. In other words, her chance of being unlucky twice in a row has now been reduced to 36 percent. Over a three-year period, if she has a third Pap smear done one year after the second, the odds are now $0.6 \times 0.6 \times .0.6 = .22$, or 22 percent. In other words, with each successive Pap test, her chances of having repeatedly false-negative Pap smears continues to decline. Eventually, in almost all cases, the lesion will be detected.

Here's where an understanding of the natural history of

dysplasia is helpful. If you recall, we learned earlier that in most women, dysplasia may take many years to progress to invasive cancer. The long incubation period means we can get away with the low sensitivity of the Pap smear, because the odds are still good that—with repeated Pap testing—the dysplasia will *still* be caught in time. In other words, the *cumulative* sensitivity of the Pap smear over time allows us to diagnose and treat almost all moderate and severe dysplasia before they progress to cancer. That's why Pap smears work as well as they do despite their low individual sensitivity, and it also explains why it's so important for women to get their Pap tests on a regular basis!

What Might Go Wrong . . .

You have some control over the accuracy of your Pap, and you can help prevent a false or unsatisfactory reading. Before you ever enter the office, you may have inadvertently affected the outcome of your Pap. Starting off the process right is vital for accuracy. Here's a list of points to remember before your examination:

Preparing for the Pap Smear

- Schedule your exam for the middle of your menstrual cycle, and *never* during your period.
- Don't use any kind of creams, douches, foams, gels, vaginal medications, or tampons for three days before your exam. They cloud the results, and anything inserted into the vagina, like a tampon, can traumatize the cervix.
- Don't have sex in the twenty-four hours before your exam—your partner's sperm can potentially mask abnormalities.

• Make sure that the laboratory evaluating your Pap smear sample is accredited by a recognized licensing body. You can call 1-800-LAB-5678 for verification.

The next step, of course, is in the hands of your doctor. More than 60 percent of false negatives occur at the point of sampling, that is, when cells are taken from your cervix. It's possible that the doctor simply didn't obtain a good sample. Another possibility is that the smear contained material such as cell debris, mucus, and bacteria that hid the abnormal cells; another is that the abnormal cells were all jumbled together and hidden under a pack of normal cells. All these things can happen, and they don't necessarily reflect poorly on the skills of your doctor.

However, even good samples can be wrongly interpreted as negative. Once the sample has made it to the lab, reading the slide is a difficult, highly skilled, and time-consuming process—the average slide holds anywhere from fifty thousand to three hundred thousand cells, but only *one* abnormal cell might indicate HSIL or cancer. So, yes, it's possible that even if you follow all the rules you're supposed to prior to the exam, and even if your doctor sends a textbook-perfect slide to the lab, you may still get a false-negative result.

Despite the training of cytotechnologists and cyto-pathologists studying your Pap smear, they *are* only human. Many doctors send their Pap smears to large commercial laboratories specializing in reading Pap smears, and these laboratories read thousands of Pap smears every year. Cytotechnologists are expected to read a certain number of slides every day, and it's possible that they might miss important abnormalities.

Most laboratories do their work very well, but a few so-called "Pap smear mills" have asked their technologists to read too many smears each day, increasing the odds of making a mistake. This kind of scenario led to scrutiny and regulation regarding the number of slides a technologist can read every day. Do mistakes still happen? Of course they do, and between inadequate sampling and misinterpretation, many women who actually have LSIL or HSIL are told they have a normal Pap smear. In other words, the Pap test is not particularly sensitive and might miss cervical disease . . . and *that's* why your doctor repeats your Pap smear on a regular basis.

False-negative Pap smears clearly pose the biggest health threat, because we could miss the cancer. At the other end of the spectrum, Pap smears may be interpreted as falsely positive. In this situation, a Pap smear might be over-interpreted and called positive when it really isn't. False positives pose a threat to your *mental* health because, until you know it's a false alarm, you'll be understandably worried!

As you know, performing and interpreting Pap smears can be a tricky business: On the one hand, we don't want to miss any serious cervical lesions; but then again, if we *over*-interpret them, they'll cause a lot of unnecessary anxiety and diagnostic tests. Fortunately, a number of recent technological advances show great promise in improving the diagnostic accuracy of Pap smears. I'll discuss these later.

False positives are a much rarer problem than false

negatives. One woman, Sarah, has had five Pap smears in the last eight years and two of these were abnormal. She believed that the abnormal Pap smears were probably both false alarms, since both of her last two follow-up Paps were normal. Unfortunately, that's backward logic—instead of believing the abnormal Paps were false positives, Sarah should have been more worried that the other Paps could have been false *negatives*. True, most mild abnormalities— about 70 percent, in fact—regress to normal within twenty-four months, but that doesn't mean she should shrug off the abnormal Pap smears as false alarms.

Newer Methods of Performing Pap Tests: Cell Suspension Methods

Fortunately, researchers constantly strive to improve the accuracy of the Pap test, including new ways to collect and prepare samples. The idea is this: Your doctor collects cells from the cervix, but instead of smearing them on slides, he or she places the cells in a small container of solution. At the lab, a special machine pulls the cells out of the solution and places them on a slide in a single cell layer. The cells don't bunch up because the machine allows only one cell in one spot. The machine also removes much of the cellular debris and mucus that hide abnormal cells in routine Pap smears. These cell "monolayers" are easier to interpret than routine Pap smears; they reduce the chances of false negatives due to inadequate samples; and they virtually eliminate common problems like cell clumping.

In addition, the machine uses only a fraction of the

cellular material in the solution. If something goes wrong in the laboratory, or the diagnosis is uncertain, the cytotechnologist can go back to the remaining material and make more monolayer slides. This extra material can also be used for HPV testing, which is performed in a variety of circumstances that are discussed later in the book.

Several companies market these solution-based Pap smear tests. One such company, the Cytyc Corporation, makes the ThinPrep test, which has been approved by the Food and Drug Administration for clinical use. Unfortunately, while this new approach offers all these advantages, it's an expensive alternative to conventional smears. Some insurance plans pay for ThinPrep, but you may have to foot the bill yourself—about forty dollars for health and peace of mind. In addition, it may not be available everywhere, even if you're willing to pay for it. The laboratory requires special processing machines to make the cell monolayers, and your doctor has to have the special collection vials on hand. Is the extra expense worth it? Probably—so you might need to do a little lobbying if at first you can't get it.

Computerized Screening of Cervical Smears

What if a computer could be designed to read Pap smears in the same way as a cytotechnologist or cytopathologist? Since they don't get tired or distracted, machines eliminate human error. In 1999, several different screening systems became available, including PAPNET and AutoPap 300 QC. These systems use neural-network-based artificial intelligence to present images of the cells with the most abnormal appearance to screeners (Bosanquet et al 1999). Note that the screeners—that is, the cytotechnologists—still play a very important role in the final interpretation of the smears. The computer picks out the abnormal Paps and puts them on a screen, and the cytotechnologist reviews the Pap. The computerized system processes the smears more quickly than humans, and this gives the screeners more time to study abnormal Paps, instead of spending too much time on normal Paps. The computerized systems don't really lead to better sensitivity, but they do improve specificity. In other words, a higher proportion of the slides initially identified as abnormal *do* have a real abnormality, and this makes the whole process more efficient. Overall, these computer systems probably won't affect the outcome of your Pap smear interpretation as much as solution-based Pap smears. The truth is, false negatives are inevitable with any method.

Polarprobe

Another emerging technology—one that's particularly exciting for both you and your doctor—is the Polarprobe. The name's a little weird, but it's a novel technology that utilizes the difference in visual and electrical properties between normal, precancerous, and cancerous cervical tissue, according to a 2000 study (Singer 2000). Squamous cells, the flat, scalelike cells protecting your cervix, are mostly uniform in size and shape, so when abnormalities occur, the cells become distorted. The Polarprobe takes advantage of those changes by emitting a combination of low-level electrical impulses and light pulses at different frequencies and wavelengths. It measures, digitizes, and compares the tissue response with a databank of cervical tissue signatures. It's kind of like deep-sea sonar, only it uses light pulses instead of sound.

The best part of the Polarprobe is its small size—about 17 centimeters long, tapering to a flat tip where the optical and electrical sensors are situated. The probe is connected to a console housing the tissue-classification software. Your doctor would insert a speculum as usual and pass the probe over your cervix for one to two minutes, and the result would be available at the end of the exam.

In other words, you can skip the whole smear-slide-ship-study process. In Singer's study, the patients responded positively because it was more comfortable than the Pap and immediate results were a big plus. In one study, the Polarprobe's sensitivity to changes in the cervix compared favorably with the Pap smear. In other words, it's just as accurate. And quicker. And less messy.

Now it's time for the caveats: This is a new technology that really hasn't been proven yet in the real world. Techniques that work well in the hands of researchers who helped develop the technique may or may not work as well in the hands of ordinary mortals. The ultimate cost of the procedure is not yet clear, and you probably won't be seeing it in your doctor's office any time soon. This isn't to say that it won't be great; it simply means that the jury is still out. So for now, we'll trust in Dr. Papanicolaou's procedure.

No method is foolproof, but they *do* keep getting better.

If your Pap smear does turn out to be abnormal, your

doctor may decide that you should have one of several follow-up diagnostic procedures, like a colposcopy or a test for HPV DNA. These procedures usually aren't recommended unless your doctor has reason to believe your Pap could advance or has advanced to dysplasia, so these procedures will be covered in chapter 6.

Get Your Pap Smear Regularly! Recommendations for Pap Smear Screening

The *only* way to be sure your cervix is in the pink is to have regular Pap smears. If your Pap *is* a false negative this time, hopefully it won't be when you go back next year. Cervical cancer can take many years to develop, so imagine how many missed Pap smears *that* takes.

> Four out of five women who die of cervical cancer did not have a Pap smear in the previous five years. (College of American Pathology)

The most common recommendation? As I said previously, women who are eighteen or sexually active—whichever comes first—should begin to have Pap smears every year (annually). Adolescent Pap screening brings up difficult issues; what teenager wants to tell her mother she needs a Pap smear because she's having sex? Parents may want to think about taking their daughters in for a gynecologic exam even earlier than eighteen, considering the possibility that a sexually active teen may not want to admit she's having sex.

The issue of administering Pap smears to young women is a hot debate these days. Most doctors would agree that Pap smears and full pelvic exams should occur with the onset of sexual activity. But how do we define *sexual activity*? A girl may believe she's a virgin because she hasn't had penetrative vaginal sex, and according to society's traditional definition, she is. But what about oral or anal intercourse? Neither are traditionally considered to be "sex," but both have their own sets of sexually transmitted diseases and issues, including HPV and herpes.

In Europe, the debate rages over whether Pap smears should be administered to women under twenty-five at all. As I said earlier, the logic is that cervical cancer rarely develops before the late twenties and early thirties, so as long as they catch it by age twenty-five, they can probably take steps to reverse the development of the cancer. Economically, it's a sensible strategy. Pap smears are expensive and since young women rarely develop cervical cancer, they save money by postponing Pap smears. Of course, that's weighing cost-effectiveness against the lives that could potentially be lost using such a strategy, a choice I certainly wouldn't want to make. My recommendation, as with any issue in this book, is education and vigilance, and to stick with current recommendations for Pap smear screening intervals until the experts tell us otherwise.

As long as a young woman is sexually active, she should be getting regular Pap smears. In fact, *all* women, even postmenopausal women, are at risk for cervical cancer, so all women should get Pap smears on a regular basis. Exams should be annual at first, but sometimes frequency can slow down to once every three years if the first three

or four specimens are normal and the woman is not considered at "high risk" for abnormal pap smears. (A list of
high-risk factors is outlined in chapter 1.)

Conclusion

In the end, your sexual health is entirely in *your* hands.
Researching and choosing a skilled doctor, getting a Pap
smear every year, understanding the process by which the
cells in your body change and grow, understanding how
your cervical cells are handled after they're collected for a
Pap test—all of these things will help you move toward a
greater control over your own health.

PART TWO

Cervical HPV

CHAPTER THREE

Unsatisfactory, Normal, and Benign Pap Smears

Now you know what a Pap smear is and how it's classified: two steps on your path to becoming an educated patient. Having bought this book, you may already have been diagnosed with an abnormal Pap smear. But for future reference, or if you're simply concerned about HPV infection, you still should know the meaning of the three lowest levels on the Bethesda scale: unsatisfactory, within normal limits, and benign cellular changes.

An "Unsatisfactory" Rating

You read in the last chapter about the accuracy of Pap tests. In general, they're a relatively trustworthy method for detecting abnormal cells. But inaccuracies occur, and that's why the Bethesda system and all previous classification systems have included an "unsatisfactory" rating. *Unsatisfactory* simply means that results are inconclusive. The most common reason is that the cytotechnologist didn't see any endocervical cells, in which case repeating the Pap or performing a colposcopy would help. The second most common reason is that the smear didn't show *enough* cells, which could either be due to doctor error—your doctor or the technician—or recent douching.

The best way to avoid an unsatisfactory rating is to follow the guidelines listed in chapter 2: In the twenty-four hours before your exam, don't have sex and don't use any creams, douches, gels, foams, or tampons, and schedule your visit for the middle of your menstrual cycle. Of course, if your doctor didn't take a large enough sample, or if something corrupted the sample at the lab, an unsatisfactory rating is beyond your control.

In either case, your doctor will probably ask you to come back to the office for another Pap smear (*sans* full pelvic examination).

"Within Normal Limits"

Hooray! "Within normal limits" is a technician's way of saying, "At the moment, you're in the clear." Some cell activity is always occurring in your cervix; as I said earlier, cells are constantly shedding, transforming, and creating a new epithelium. But "within normal limits" should indicate that the cell activity is normal, with no infections or abnormalities present. For a look at a healthy, "normal" Pap smear, see figure 2.2.

Keep in mind, though, that what your doctor tells you and what the test reveals may occasionally be two different things. When a Pap comes back with very mild abnormalities (covered in the next chapter), sometimes your doctor may tell you you're fine anyway. After all, most abnormal Paps regress to normal within six months.

The problem with this logic is threefold: First, you're not getting the whole story from your doctor. Perhaps, if you knew slight abnormalities existed in your Pap, you could change some of your habits to strengthen your immune system—nutrition and smoking play roles in the health of your cervix. And most women *I* know would like to know if something's not 100 percent right, no matter how small it is.

Second, what if three successive Paps have come back mildly abnormal? Mild abnormalities alone are usually not cause for panic, but consistently abnormal Paps could indicate a deeper problem. In this case, a slightly abnormal Pap could advance to LSIL and HSIL, more serious conditions covered in chapters 5 and 6.

Finally, and most important, a chance always exists that you may not go back for your Pap in a year. In any case, you should always have your annual Pap smear and pelvic exam, but what if you move to a different city and have a new doctor? He or she will ask for your health history, and you won't know that your previous Pap showed slight abnormalities.

Ask your doctor for all the details. Clearly, trust between you and your doctor is of vital importance, a topic I cover in appendix A. You should have an open relationship with your doctor and feel free to question him or her for your own peace of mind.

Keep in mind, too, that a normal Pap smear doesn't rule out the possibility of HPV infection. Many women have HPV and never show any symptoms of it, just as many women treated for an advanced stage of HPV infection, like dysplasia, can have normal Pap smears forever after. HPV itself is not necessarily cured. Finally, you should also remember that a normal Pap smear doesn't necessarily exclude dysplasia—for the reasons we already discussed, Pap smears have limited sensitivity and might miss lesions. Regular annual Pap smears are therefore essential for your continued sexual health.

"Benign Cellular Changes"

Here, *benign* means "noncancerous" changes, not changes that aren't potentially harmful to your health. A Pap test, along with identifying abnormal cellular activity, can also pinpoint infections unrelated to HPV or cancerous changes. These infections should be treated, and your doctor will probably prescribe treatment for you.

Following is a list of infections that can lead to a diagnosis of "benign cellular changes" on a Pap smear.

Yeast Infections

If you haven't had a yeast infection, you probably know someone who has—75 percent of all women will experience at least one vaginal yeast infection in their lives, and recurring infections are common. Yeast infections are not cause for great alarm, but any woman who's had one will tell you they're unpleasant.

Symptoms

Common symptoms of yeast infections include itching, burning, dryness, redness, and irritation of the vaginal area. Advanced infection can also cause vulvar swelling and painful urination. Vaginal discharge is usually thick, whitish, and cottage-cheese–like.

Cause

Yeast infections are usually caused by *Candida albicans*, a yeast fungus naturally found in your mouth, vagina, and intestinal tract. It's always there, but your body's natural chemistry controls the fungus. When the yeast multiplies beyond your body's ability to control it, you develop the signs and symptoms of a yeast infection. One factor that protects your cervix and vagina from developing symptoms of a yeast infection is the so-called "good" bacteria in your vagina. These bacteria maintain a good acid-base balance in the vagina and help to protect the cervical and vaginal epithelium from the yeast. Some of the more common of these bacteria are known as *lactobacilli*.

When the good bacteria can no longer provide balance, the yeast may grow out of control. As you may know, antibiotics often throw off your body's "good" bacteria in addition to killing whatever "bad" bacteria you were taking the antibiotics for (for instance, *streptococci* in strep throat). Women who have diabetes suffer from more frequent vaginal yeast infections than women with normal blood sugar. In addition, wearing nylon or Lycra underwear traps moisture and heat, providing the yeast with an ideal setting for growth. Other contributing factors include obesity, the use of oral contraceptives, and loss of immunity through pregnancy.

Treatment

If it's your first yeast infection, your doctor will probably suggest medication for you, usually in the form of suppositories and cream. Most doctors recommend using the seven-day, or at least three-day, over-the-counter treatments. The one-day treatments are convenient but rarely kill off all of the infection—which means it'll be back in a week or so. In addition, a prescription pill called Diflucan, taken once, can cure a yeast infection in five days, but in the meantime, creams soothe the itching and discomfort.

Keep in mind that most vaginal creams contain oils, so condoms may *not* be effective during usage of these creams (the latex in condoms has a tendency to break down in the presence of different kinds of oil). In general, sexual intercourse is a bad idea if you have a bad yeast infection; not only is sex uncomfortable and even painful, but sex can aggravate an infection and even transmit the infection to your partner. Some doctors treat partners, particularly when the woman has a history of multiple recurrences despite treatment.

Dozens of over-the-counter products cure yeast infections, but don't self-treat unless you've had a previous infection and are sure of the diagnosis. Many women mistake bacterial vaginosis for yeast infections, and gone untreated, bacterial vaginosis can contribute to more serious conditions such as pelvic inflammatory disease.

Prevention

As with most cervical and vaginal infections, an ounce of prevention is worth a pound of cure. If you're on antibiotics, you may find eating a cup of yogurt with active bacteria a day or taking daily doses of acidophilus supplements helpful. Cotton panties, preferably white, allow your genitals to "breathe." You should also avoid bubble baths and feminine powders and sprays if you're prone to yeast infections, and *never* douche. Douching removes your body's protective layer of mucus and leaves your vagina and cervix vulnerable to infection. And practice safe sex! Condoms help prevent STDs and other vaginal infections.

Bacterial vaginosis and cervicitis

Cervicitis simply means "inflammation of the cervix," so technically, it refers to any infection in the cervix and can also coexist with dysplasia (covered in the next chapter). But a mild form of cervicitis can be caused by untreated *bacterial vaginosis.* In fact, many women who believe they have yeast infections actually have this condition, which can contribute to the development of the more serious pelvic inflammatory disease (PID).

Symptoms

The symptoms of bacterial vaginosis are less obvious than yeast infections—an unpleasant, fishy odor and, occasionally but not always, an itching or burning sensation.

Cause

Like yeast infections, bacterial vaginosis is associated with loss of the normal bacteria that inhabit and protect the vagina, such as *lactobacilli*. There's often an overgrowth of anaerobic bacteria (bacteria that live in the absence of oxygen) and a particular bacterium known as *Gardnerella vaginalis*, which usually exists in small numbers in the vagina.

Bacterial vaginosis occurs most during the reproductive years, although any woman is susceptible. Risk increases with menopause, diabetes, and decreased immunity. Other contributing factors include hot weather, poor general health and hygiene, use of an intrauterine device for birth control, and douching.

Because the symptoms are so subtle, you may not realize you have bacterial vaginosis until it shows up in your Pap smear, or you might misdiagnose it and treat for a yeast infection. That's another reason why you shouldn't douche—douching before a pelvic exam masks the signs of infection.

Treatment

Treatment is simple and effective. Your doctor can prescribe Cleocin 2 percent vaginal cream, a three-to-seven-night treatment, or oral antibiotics such as metronidazole (trade name is Flagyl).

Note, however, that antibiotics themselves can lead to yeast infections, and there is a risk of back-to-back vaginal infections.

Prevention

Always wipe from front to back after a bowel move-ment. Keep your vaginal area clean and dry, and some doc-tors even recommend washing before and after sex with an antibacterial cleanser. Avoid tight clothing and, again, wear white cotton panties. Personal hygiene products, spermi-cides, harsh soaps, and detergents should also be avoided if you have particular sensitivity to them. As for birth con-trol, always wash your diaphragm, cervical cap, or medica-tion applicator after each use.

Genital Herpes

Like human papillomaviruses, herpes simplex virus (HSV) is a common sexually transmitted virus, so common that some say it's the STD "everybody has but no one talks about." And now you know that HPV fits perfectly into that category, too! And although forty-five million people are in-fected with HSV (80 percent of whom are not aware of their infection, since they don't develop symptoms or don't recognize them when they occur), everybody does *not* have it. So you can help slow the HSV epidemic.

Symptoms

Though symptoms often depend on the person's im-munity and sensitivity, the initial breakout usually appears within two to ten days after first infection and lasts up to two to three weeks. Early symptoms include an itching or burning sensation, pain in the legs, buttocks, or genital area, vaginal discharge, and a feeling of pressure in the ab-domen. A few days later, sores or lesions may erupt at the site of the infection, usually in the vagina, cervix, or urinary tract of women, and in the urinary tract or penis of men. Herpes lesions first appear as small red bumps, which develop into blisters with clear fluid inside them. These then become painful, open sores, then heal without scarring. The first episode—which is usually the worst—can also include a fever, headache, muscle aches, urinary pain or difficulty, and swollen glands in the groin area.

After the initial episode, HSV travels from the infection site to sensory nerves and then along those nerves to the end of the spinal cord, where it remains inside the nerve cells in an inactive or dormant state. Most of the time, HSV remains that way and does not cause too many other problems. In some cases, the virus reactivates often, such as monthly, traveling back to the site of the original lesion and causing new sores. Often menstruation, stress, and other infections such as colds can trigger an episode. HSV *can* reactivate without any sores or lesions, and during these "invisible" recurrences, small amounts of HSV can shed from around the initial breakout site.

Herpes is usually simple to diagnose but occasionally it can be difficult. Some physicians may attribute the red bumps to ingrown hairs or an allergic reaction. If you have *any* suspicion that herpes could be the culprit, ask your doctor to conduct the necessary tests (usually a virus culture obtained from swabbing an open sore).

Cause

Herpes is caused by the herpes simplex virus. Two types of herpes exist, and both kinds affect the genitals *and* the mouth. However, HSV 1 usually occurs on the lips in the form of fever blisters and cold sores. HSV 2 most commonly appears in the genitals. Both types of herpes can reactivate at any point in a person's lifetime.

Treatment

Although three drugs currently exist to treat the symptoms of genital herpes, they can only reduce the severity and frequency of recurrent episodes as well as shorten the length of first episodes. *They are not cures.* Zovirax (acyclovir), Famvir (famcyclovir), and Valtrex (valacyclovir) are all approved to treat both first and recurrent episodes.

Prevention

Transmission of herpes can occur during any active period, whether sores appear or not—which means that the genital secretions and imperceptible lesions can also transmit the virus. In addition, herpes can be transmitted through oral sex. If your partner has a cold sore in his or her mouth and performs oral sex on you, you could get genital herpes. Or if you have genital herpes and your partner performs oral sex on you, you could transmit it to his or her mouth. If there's *any* chance that you or your partner has oral herpes or genital herpes, refrain from oral sex or use a condom or "dental dam" (a square piece of latex for use in female oral sex or for oral-anal sex). Keep in mind that like HPV, HSV is spread by skin-to-skin contact, so you could still transmit it outside of the area covered by the condom.

Keep the infected area clean and dry; don't touch the sores (wash your hands immediately if you do); and refrain from sex from the time of the appearance of the first symptoms until the sores are healed and covered with new skin.

Condoms offer some protection between active episodes, but again, because HSV's transmitted by skin-to-skin contact, condoms may not cover all infected areas. The best route is to discuss the possibility of transmission with your partner and use condoms.

Complications

In addition to the uncomfortable outward symptoms of herpes, other health complications can arise. *Always* tell any new doctor that you have genital HSV. Weakened immune systems can cause severe and long-lasting episodes. Pregnant women should be especially careful—if the first episode occurs during pregnancy, they can pass the virus on to their babies and may be at a higher risk for premature delivery. About half of babies born with HSV die or suffer neurological damage; they can develop encephalitis, severe rashes, and eye problems. (The drug acyclovir improves the outcome for many babies, which is why your obstetrician needs to know.) During active infection at the time of delivery, cesarean section is usually recommended, especially for a mother who's having her first outbreak of herpes; between outbreaks, the risk of transmission to your baby through vaginal birth is very low.

If you don't have HSV, my recommendation is simple: Always use condoms, and make sure you know your partner's sexual history *before* having sex. If you have herpes, be vigilant about taking proper care of the symptoms during episodes, and discuss your condition with past and present sexual partners.

Trichomonas Infection

Trichomonas is a common but little-known sexually transmitted infection caused by a little bug called *Trichomonas vaginalis,* a protozoan that can take up residence in a woman's vagina and cervix or in a man's urinary tract. About three million women are infected annually, but some estimate that 30 to 50 percent of all women may be infected with trichomonas at some point. The proportion of men with trichomonas is unknown.

Symptoms

Unfortunately, trichomonas is often asymptomatic, especially in men, so many people don't know they're infected. About four to twenty days after infection, women may experience vaginal irritation or itching, vaginal inflammation, painful intercourse, and thin, odorous yellowish, greenish, or white discharge. Diagnosis is difficult in men (usually swabbing the urethra is the only option), and most of women's infections are found during a pelvic exam and Pap smear.

Treatment and Prevention

Trichomonas is curable, usually with Flagyl (metronidazole). Some doctors treat partners as well to prevent reinfection, particularly when there is a history of multiple recurrence. Although trichomonas is usually sexually transmitted and can be prevented by using condoms, it can also be transmitted by dirty towels and washcloths, so make sure not to share those items. As with other vaginal bacterial infections, white cotton panties are recommended.

Conclusion

The above list of things that can cause "benign changes" is by no means all-inclusive. Although the purpose of the Pap smear is to diagnose cervical LSIL and HSIL associated with HPV, Pap smears can often diagnose these other infections. If your Pap smear is classified as "benign changes" and shows signs of one of those other infections such as bacterial vaginosis, your doctor would probably call to tell you that you have bacterial vaginosis, rather than say you have an abnormal Pap smear. Follow-up diagnostic procedures are required for some of these infections such as HSV, and, as I said before, the presence of these diseases does *not* mean you don't have HPV.

If you're unsure about anything in your Pap smear, or you have reason to believe that you may be at risk for an STD, tell your doctor.

Tips to Help You Avoid Infection

STDs: The Three Cs

- **Condoms, condoms, condoms!** While not foolproof, condoms greatly decrease your risk of transmitting an STD and developing bacterial infections of the cervix and vagina. You know this. Your partner knows this. Use them!
- **Communication.** Talk to your partner if you have a sexually transmitted disease, so that you can make a decision together regarding protection. Not saying anything and depending on condom use is not fair to either of you—and especially unfair to the people who may get it because your partner doesn't know he or she may have it. It's a tough discussion, but well worth it.

- **Common sense.** Be careful who you choose as your sexual partner. It's as simple as that. Know your partner's sexual history before engaging in sexual activity, whether it's vaginal, anal, or oral intercourse. *You're worth it.*

Prevention of vaginal bacterial infections

- **Don't douche!** Let me say this again: Don't douche! Your genitals are self-cleansing, and whether you experience a heavy or a light discharge on a daily basis, that discharge is good for you. The mucous membrane lining the cervix and vagina cleans and protects your vagina, and without it, you're susceptible to a host of infections. In addition, douching can mask symptoms, which will only make an infection last longer.
- **Wear cotton underwear.** It sounds silly and simple, but wearing white cotton underwear—or underwear with at least a cotton panel—will go a long way in letting your genitals "breathe." Nylon holds in moisture and heat, and there's nothing bacteria love more than a warm, dark, wet place for breeding.
- **Practice good hygiene.** Keep the area clean and dry, and try washing with an antibacterial soap. Don't borrow anyone's dirty towels or washcloths, and wash out any reuseable applicators, cervical caps, and diaphragms after each use.
- **Boost your immunity.** General wellness will increase your body's ability to fight off infection. So eat a balanced diet, keep your weight within healthy limits, and don't smoke (but you already knew that, didn't you?).
- **Avoid using perfumed products like bubble bath, bath oils, powders, feminine deodorant sprays, and harsh detergents.** A bubble bath once in a while is fine, but if you're particularly sensitive, try to avoid them altogether.
- **Use condoms.** Again, condoms reduce the risk of transmitting bacterial and viral infections, either to or from your partner.

Questions to Ask Your Doctor

Unsatisfactory

- When should I come in for my repeat Pap?
- What may have caused the unsatisfactory rating?

Normal

- When should I come in for my next Pap?
- So my Pap didn't show any abnormalities at all?

Benign Changes

- What treatment do you recommend for [the infection]?
- How did I get the infection?
- How can I avoid getting it again?
- Does my partner need to be examined?
- Should I come in for a follow-up exam regarding the infection?
- When should I come in for my next Pap?

CHAPTER FOUR

Abnormal Paps:
An ASCUS Diagnosis

You've done what every woman should do: You went to your doctor for your annual exam—Pap smear, breast exam, the works. Afterward, you went home or returned to work and promptly forgot all about the ten minutes in the stirrups.

Two weeks later, a nurse calls you and says your Pap smear had some abnormalities in it. If you know what abnormalities *could* indicate, you might panic and think they indicate cancer; if you're not sure what the Pap smear indicates, maybe you just figure it's another yeast infection. In almost all cases, having an abnormal Pap smear doesn't mean you have cancer, but as you know, they're not to be taken lightly, either. An attitude of cautious concern would do well for you here. By all means, don't panic, but don't blow it off, either. Since you bought this book, I'll assume you've already been diagnosed with an abnormal Pap smear or you know someone who has.

So What *Does* ASCUS Indicate?

ASCUS, which stands for Atypical Squamous Cell changes of Undetermined Significance, is a designation specifically created by the Bethesda system (the system for classifying Pap smears described in chapter 2). This diagnosis is used if a cytotechnologist or cytopathologist notes changes that are more suspicious than "benign changes," but the changes don't meet all of the criteria for low-grade lesions or high-grade lesions. Since the meaning of these changes is not clear, the Pap smear result is deemed to be of "undetermined significance."

But life is more complicated than that. In fact, ASCUS is divided into two categories: ASC-US (unsatisfactory significance) and ASC-H (cells that cannot exclude HSIL). If the category is ASC-US, that means your cells show some increased activity, but you're unlikely to have HSIL. In this case, your doctor will probably adopt the wait-and-see attitude: "Come back in three to six months and we'll see if anything's changed." They may also perform an HPV test, which, if positive, would lead to colposcopy. If the HPV test is negative, then the Pap could be repeated in three to six months. Some doctors, though, might even go straight to colposcopy.

If your Pap is diagnosed as ASC-H, many doctors will immediately perform a colposcopy, since it may indicate the presence of HSIL.

In general, ASCUS isn't a precancerous change; it just indicates some cellular change that *could* develop into dysplasia. ASCUS could even reflect the presence of existing dysplasia. If you have a history of STDs, HPV in particular, you should tell your doctor anyway, but if your Pap comes back with an ASCUS label, don't hesitate to give him or her information about your sexual health history.

A diagnosis of ASCUS means something *might or might not* be wrong with respect to HPV or dysplasia. It could also indicate the presence of one or more of the infections that we covered in the previous chapter. Part of the workup of an ASCUS Pap smear might include diagnostic tests for the presence of candida infection, bacterial vaginosis, or trichomonas. If one or more of these infections are present, your Pap will probably return to normal after treatment.

Here's the good news: Most of the time, an ASCUS diagnosis regresses to normal by the time of the follow-up Pap smear.

Here's a chart of results of sequential Pap smears to give you an idea of how often this occurs:

Abnormal Class	Regression to Normal	Progression to Higher Grade over 24 Months	Progression to Invasive Cancer over 24 Months
ASCUS	68%	7%	0.25%
LSIL	47%	21%	0.15%
HSIL	35%	23%	1.44%

Source: Women's Diagnostic Cyber, *www.dxcyber.com.*

As you can see, most ASCUS Pap smears do return to normal. That can mean one of three things: Your body fought off the infection that made your Pap smear abnormal; the original Pap smear was a false positive; or the follow-up Pap smear is a false negative.

To summarize, three follow-up options have been proposed for women with an ASCUS diagnosis: Repeat the Pap test, undergo immediate colposcopy, or undergo testing for the presence of HPV itself. If your Pap shows ASC-US, any of these three options would be reasonable. If your Pap shows ASC-H, though, you'll probably have a colposcopy.

Colposcopy

As I said before, you may be referred for a colposcopy because your Pap smear was abnormal. Why? Because the Pap smear is basically a jumble of cells on a slide. If some are abnormal, your doctor can't tell where those cells came from in the cervicovaginal tract. Furthermore, the Pap smear isn't reliable enough by itself to determine the level of severity of the cervical disease, and the level of severity will determine whether or not you receive treatment. So if your doctor thinks your abnormal Pap smear deserves further workup, he or she will want a pathologist to microscopically inspect a sample of your tissue.

Your doctor obtains that tissue sample (called a biopsy) by performing a colposcopy, in which he or she visualizes the lesion through the colposcope and samples the suspicious area. A colposcopy is a short, in-office procedure that involves both a visual examination of the cervix, vagina, and vulva, and taking a biopsy of the abnormal area for microscopic examination by the pathologist. Colposcopy is a specialized procedure, and performance of this technique requires extensive training and certification. The whole process takes about ten to fifteen minutes.

First, your doctor inserts the vaginal speculum. Next, he or she uses a colposcope, a large, electric microscope positioned about 30 centimeters from your vagina. A picture of a colposcope is shown in figure 4.1. A bright light on the end of it illuminates your cervix. Often the colposcope will project an image onto a television screen so that you, too, can see your cervix. The purpose of colposcopy is to rule out cancer and find the most severe form of dysplasia possible, since that guides treatment.

Doctors use several tricks to increase the sensitivity of colposcopy and identify the most severe areas of abnormality. First, they use 5 percent acetic acid, better known as vinegar. Yep—vinegar! In the presence of the vinegar, areas of dysplasia will appear to be white through the colposcope, a process called acetowhitening. Dysplasia can be quite subtle or missed altogether in the absence of the vinegar or the colposcopic magnification.

The next trick is to use a green filter for the colposcope light. A series of criteria guide the doctor toward the worst areas of disease. These include the appearance and organization of blood vessels on the cervix, and these patterns become more visible under the green light. Since cells in the lesion grow so much faster than normal cells, they need extra blood and nutrition, which causes abnormal blood vessel growth into the lesion.

Some of these patterns show up as pinpoint red dots,

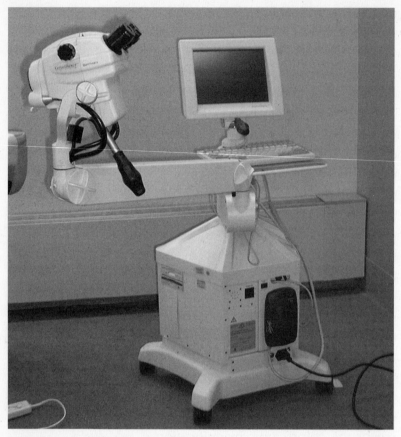

Figure 4.1: A Colposcope. *This figure shows a colposcope. Once the vaginal speculum (fig. 2.3) is inserted, the colposcope is rolled up to the opening of the speculum. After the 5 percent acetic acid is applied, the walls of the cervix, vagina, and vulva are examined with the magnification provided by the colposcope. (Author's photo.)*

known as *vascular punctation*. Another pattern is called *vascular mosaicism*, since the blood vessels are found in a mosaic pattern. Other features of the lesions that will be noted by the colposcopists will be the surface characteristics. Is the lesion flat or bumpy (*papillary* in medicalese)?

Is it smooth or granular in appearance? Is the surface of the skin broken or ulcerated—often signs of invasive cancer?

Finally, colposcopists may apply Lugol's solution, an iodine-based concoction that has the opposite effect of vinegar on dysplasia. With the vinegar, normal cervical tissue usually doesn't change color. With Lugol's solution, the normal tissues turn a deep brown color while the lesions tend to turn a pale yellow or stay white. The more severe the lesion, the less the Lugol's uptake. Using all of these methods, the colposcopist will decide which if any of these areas need to be biopsied. Figure 2.3 shows what dysplasia looks like on the cervix when seen through the colposcope.

To take a biopsy, the colposcopist uses an instrument called a forceps, a sharp pincer that grabs a small piece of tissue. These are shown in figure 2.5. After taking the tissue, the doctor drops it into a preservative called formalin and then sends it for examination by the pathologist. The biopsy can be slightly painful, so taking two ibuprofen or acetaminophen beforehand could curb the pain. Your doctor will probably give you a sanitary napkin afterward, and you might experience light spotting while the areas of biopsy heal. To speed healing, don't have sex or use tampons or any creams, douches, etc., for several days following the colposcopy.

Endocervical Curettage

For colposcopy to be considered successful, your doctor must be able to view the entire lesion. If he or she can't see the entire lesion, the colposcopy is considered "unsatisfactory." If part of the lesion is in your endocervical canal, it may not be completely visible, and the doctor will have to perform an endocervical curettage (ECC). In this case, he or she will use a curette, a small, spoon-shaped instrument, to scrape tissue from inside the endocervical canal for biopsy. ECCs are necessary in 10 to 20 percent of women and they're more commonly required by older women.

If an ECC shows abnormal cells but your doctor can't see the entire lesion, then he or she will usually recommend a treatment procedure called a cone biopsy, described later in this book. Your doctor wants to be able to rule out invasive cancer, and the only way to do that is to remove the suspicious matter for examination under the microscope.

Dilatation and Curettage (D&C)

In the event that it's not clear whether an abnormal Pap test or your symptoms are caused by problems in the cervix or by problems higher up in the endometrium (the lining of the uterus), your doctor may perform a procedure called a *dilatation and curettage*, also known as a D&C. Unlike a routine cervical biopsy, D&Cs require anesthesia. This can usually be performed in-office or in a hospital. The "dilatation" part simply means your doctor stretches your cervical opening. The "curettage" part means he or she will use a curette to scrape tissue from the lining of the uterus and from the endocervical canal. The procedure may cause some bleeding and pain, and in general, the healing is similar to cervical biopsy.

Testing for HPV and How the HPV Test Is Different from the Pap Smear: The Hybrid Capture II HPV DNA Test

So far, I've told you about how HPV contributes to the development of dysplasia and cancer, and how the Pap smear can be used to detect early signs of dysplasia and cancer. Since HPV is so important in these diseases, can we test for HPV to diagnose dysplasia and cancer? The answer is "maybe" and this is the basis of the one HPV test approved by the Food and Drug Administration for clinical use—the Hybrid Capture II (HC-II) test, made by the Digene Corporation. Distinguishing between the HPV test and the Pap test can be a little confusing, so let me digress a little to remind you how they are different: The Pap test examines cervical and vaginal cells for cellular changes that indicate the presence of dysplasia or cancer. On the other hand, the HPV test looks directly for the virus that *causes* these changes. Instead of looking for changes in the cells, which is what the Pap test does, the HPV test looks for HPV DNA and RNA that may be present in those cells.

How Can Having an HPV Test Help When Your Pap Smear Shows ASCUS?

Clearly the HPV test and the Pap test look for different things. Can the HPV test be of any value in women who are having a Pap test? If you have a diagnosis of ASCUS, the answer seems to be yes. As I said earlier, an ASCUS diagnosis could indicate a more advanced level of dysplasia. HPV testing could help to distinguish women with ASCUS and a true HPV-related lesion from women with ASCUS not related to cancer-causing HPV infection. Rather than bringing you back to the office for another Pap smear or for colposcopy, the laboratory can use a part of a ThinPrep sample to test for the presence of HPV DNA.

> Note: No reliable *blood* test can tell you if you were previously exposed to HPV or if you currently have cervical HPV infection. The only reliable way to detect cervical HPV infection is to look directly for the HPV DNA in cervical samples.

How Does Knowing If You Have HPV Help?

If your doctor used the ThinPrep method of Pap preparation, the Hybrid Capture test can be performed on the remaining cells—the cells left *after* cells are removed for the Pap smear. In this case, you won't need to return to the office to have another sample taken. On the other hand, if you had a conventional Pap smear on a glass slide, these cells can't be used for HPV testing and you'll need to return to the office to provide another sample.

The Hybrid Capture test doesn't tell you which HPV type you have. Instead, it tests for a group of the high-risk cancer-causing HPV types together in a cocktail. If your test is positive, you might have any one of these types—or possibly more than one of them. It really doesn't matter if you don't know which one(s) you have; they all put you at risk of cancer. A nononcogenic version is also available; it detects the common non-cancer-causing HPV types such as HPV 6 or 11. (Most of the time, the laboratory doesn't perform this version of the test, since we're more concerned with the HPV types that cause cancer.)

If the Hybrid Capture test indicates that you have a cancer-causing type of HPV, then that probably means you have a higher risk of having true dysplasia, not just "atypical" cells. Since your doctor knows you're at risk for more serious conditions such as severe dysplasia and cervical cancer, he or she will probably recommend colposcopy to thoroughly examine your cervix and take a biopsy for further testing.

If your Hybrid Capture test shows you don't have a cancer-causing HPV type, then the ASCUS diagnosis could have been caused by several scenarios. A low-risk HPV type could cause the ASCUS changes. Maybe the ASCUS is due to one of the other infections that we discussed. Or the ASCUS might have been a false-positive test. In any case, you'll be asked back for a follow-up Pap in a few months. Make that appointment and keep it!

Just to reiterate one more time: When your doctor performs a Pap test, he or she is looking for changes in the cells that are caused by HPV, but is not looking for the virus itself. On the other hand, when a test like Hybrid Capture is performed, the doctor searches directly for the virus. Say you get hives on your arm—think of that as the "Pap test." It's a visible abnormality. Doing a specific allergy test to find out what caused the hives—that's the Hybrid Capture-II.

HPV testing is still in its early stage, but results have been encouraging so far: For women with ASCUS, using a combination of the ThinPrep test and Hybrid Capture, doctors can identify who is most at risk for dysplasia.

Some debate still rages, though, on the most appropriate use of the Hybrid Capture test in other settings. Its use in the setting of ASCUS is reasonably well established. But other women—women who don't have ASCUS—may also ask for HPV testing. These usually include (1) women who don't necessarily show dysplasia but who think they may have HPV; and (2) women who know they have dysplasia and want to know if they're at risk for cervical cancer. Let's deal with each of these scenarios separately.

A sexually active woman who knows she's at high risk of HPV exposure may wonder if she carries the virus herself, and the only way to answer that question would be to perform the HPV test. Sounds like a logical thing to do, right?

The answer is "Yes . . . and no." Some studies, particularly of women at high risk of dysplasia, have shown that the HPV test is actually better than the Pap smear at identifying a woman who has severe dysplasia—not a difficult feat, as you now know. So HPV testing, along with Pap smears, could actually be useful for screening high-risk women to reduce the risk of a false-negative Pap smear. That's the good news for HPV testing. Although that's not really why the woman asked for the test.

The bad news is that in other clinical settings, such as a generally healthy, relatively low-risk population, the HPV test will identify women with severe dysplasia, but a much higher proportion of the women with positive HPV tests show no signs of cervical disease at all. Remember, women can shed the virus in the absence of detectable disease. Put differently, in a generally healthy, low-risk population, most of the positive HPV tests will be found in women who have no signs of cervical disease. Your doctor will end up telling you that you have HPV, but he or she can't do anything since there's no treatment for HPV itself—only for the lesions that it causes.

We don't really know what the significance is of having a positive HPV test when you don't have a lesion—in many, if not most cases, dysplasia never occurs and follow-up HPV tests will be negative. Basically, we can't do much about the result of the test, and you'll worry for nothing. On the other hand, it's possible that some HPV-positive, disease-free women may develop HPV-associated disease later. Or they may have had a false-negative Pap smear. We simply don't know.

At some point in the future, HPV testing may assume a more prominent role in screening. One potentially interesting use of the HPV test is for women over the age of thirty. Think back to figure 1.4, which shows that most women get their HPV infection soon after initiating sexual activity but have negative HPV tests by the time they reach age thirty. The women who remain positive for HPV after thirty are probably at the highest risk of developing severe dysplasia and cervical cancer.

For screening purposes, restricting the HPV test to women over the age of thirty might make sense (European doctors are trying this approach now). Here's the idea: If you're over thirty and have a cancer-causing HPV type, you should probably have a more thorough examination. On the other hand, if your HPV test is negative, you probably won't run into problems, so you can increase the interval of your Pap smears. Some doctors in Europe are recommending Pap smear screening every five years, or even longer, for women over the age of thirty with a negative HPV test. We're not ready to make that recommendation here in the United States, but stay tuned as more information on the safety of this approach comes in over the next few years.

I don't think HPV testing will be used for screening or to replace Pap smears in the near future. That may change as more studies come in. But for now, most doctors recommend sticking with the Pap smear, "warts and all," since we know that it usually does the job.

Now let's return to the second scenario: the woman who we *know* has dysplasia. She wants to know if she's at risk for cervical cancer. If she has mild dysplasia, it'll probably go away by itself without treatment. In a recent large study, almost all of the mild lesions were caused by a cancer-causing HPV type—and then they regressed spontaneously! So if you have mild dysplasia, knowing that you have a cancer-causing HPV type isn't all that useful. Regardless of the HPV result, your doctor will follow up with another Pap to see if the lesion goes away without treatment.

Now suppose that you know that you have moderate or severe dysplasia. Would knowing that you have a cancer-causing, high-risk HPV type be helpful? Not really, because almost *all* of these lesions have oncogenic HPV types, and your doctor will treat you regardless of any HPV result. If you have itching or burning due to poison ivy, knowing which particular poison ivy plant you were exposed to isn't going to change your treatment. So, once again, the information provided by the HPV test won't help you much.

What about men? Unfortunately for men, we can't easily collect a sample from the penis for the Hybrid Capture test, so HPV testing of the penis is not an option at all at this time. To obtain an adequate number of cells for examination, the area must be moist—which is fine for the cervix or anus, but penis skin is too dry for a sufficient sample. For men, a "vinegar" test with magnification (covered in chapter 14) is the best method to look for HPV-related lesions on the penis.

To summarize, HPV testing definitely has a place in today's management of dysplasia. If you have an ASCUS diagnosis, the HPV test can determine if you need immediate colposcopy or just a repeat Pap smear. Another future use may be to screen women in conjunction with a Pap smear, but most doctors would say that we don't have enough information to recommend that yet.

Recurrent ASCUS Diagnosis on a Pap Smear

As I mentioned before, if your second or third follow-up Pap also indicates ASCUS, further diagnostic procedures such as colposcopy will determine the severity of your problem. But what if you've had an ASCUS before, such as ten years ago? Or you were treated for dysplasia years ago, your Pap smear was normal for many years, and then your Pap smear shows ASCUS this time?

You and your doctor can decide together how to deal with an ASCUS result on a Pap smear "after the fact." If you've already been treated for moderate or severe dysplasia, then you know you have HPV, so you know you're at risk for cervical cancer. Should you immediately advance to colposcopy or watch and wait? Again, if your most recent Pap also shows an ASCUS diagnosis, you might want to consider colposcopy—you may have hidden lesions that could advance to cancer. If you'd prefer to avoid any invasive procedures immediately, you'll at least want to return for a repeat Pap. But in the meantime, perhaps just examining your lifestyle and determining other contributing factors will guide you toward a healthy diagnosis. (If you're pregnant, have acquired an immunity disorder, or are taking immunosuppressants, those are possible causes for a recurrence. Other possible reasons are poor nutrition and smoking.)

Pregnancy and ASCUS

Why are you at increased risk of developing ASCUS (or any other Pap smear abnormality) if you're pregnant? The answer's simple: Pregnancy is a state of immunosuppression, and as you've already learned, immunosuppressed people are at increased risk of developing HPV-related lesions.

OK, so why is pregnancy a state of immunosuppression? Basically, when you carry a baby, you're carrying a little person who's half you and half someone else. Your immune system doesn't like to see anything but yourself, and it's trained to seek and destroy anything that isn't "you." So basically, while you're pregnant, your immune system is taking a bit of a vacation—not a *complete* vacation, but a vacation—so that it doesn't hurt the part of your child that gets its genes from its father.

While you're pregnant, your immune system may not function as well as it does normally, and you might be prone to more or longer colds, for example. You're also prone to a reactivation or worsening of your HPV infection if you already have one—you might develop a newly abnormal Pap smear or genital warts. That's the bad news. The good news is, after you deliver, your immune system rapidly returns to normal, and many of these problems resolve themselves.

So if you're pregnant and you develop ASCUS, my advice to you is simple: Get follow-up Pap smears, especially postpartum. You may need a colposcopy. If your doctor doesn't suspect cervical cancer, then he or she will likely advise a wait-and-see approach. In any case, it's critical that you return for your follow-up exams, since your postpartum recovery will determine how your further workup and care will proceed.

Atypical Glandular Cells of Undetermined Significance (AGUS)

Another condition that may appear on your Pap smear is AGUS: Abnormal *Glandular* cells of Undetermined Significance. The condition is rare, occurring in less than 1 percent of all Pap smears. While ASCUS *may* indicate more serious problems, AGUS often *does* indicate more serious problems. Abnormal glandular cells suggest the presence of potential adenocarcinoma, rather than the more common squamous cell carcinoma. (Cervical cancer is usually squamous cell cancer, while adenocarcinoma could indicate endometrial [uterine] cancer or cancer of the glands of the endocervical canal.)

AGUS is considered a "gray area" pathologically. It could indicate severe dysplasia in the glandular cells; or it could just indicate an overactive cell change. (Ronnett et al. 1999) Because 20 to 50 percent of women with AGUS have a more severe, hidden lesion, your doctor should treat this condition more aggressively than ASCUS. AGUS less frequently regresses to normal.

Usually, a pathologist will diagnose AGUS as "favor reactive"—that is, more likely to be overactive cell changes—or "favor neoplasia"—cells that probably indicate more serious abnormalities. These resemble the ASCUS designations of ASC-US and ASC-H, respectively. While a "favor reactive" diagnosis is more common, a "favor neoplasia" suggests that a precancerous condition may already have developed. In "AGUS favor neoplasia," a follow-up colposcopy will often show dysplasia. That's why follow-up is so important.

Therefore, I would recommend an immediate colposcopy for both forms of AGUS, as well as endocervical curettage (both are described earlier in this chapter). If any hidden lesions exist, your doctor can then move on to treatment procedures such as LEEP and conization (covered in chapter 6).

Conclusion

An ASCUS Pap can be frustrating for you and your doctor. So many questions arise with an uncertain diagnosis: Should we treat it? Do I need an HPV test? Should I wait for another Pap? How long should I live with ASCUS before having some other diagnostic procedure? Hopefully I've answered your questions, but above all, make sure that you return for your repeat Pap smears when recommended. They could save your life.

Topics to Discuss with Your Doctor

Tell Your Doctor . . .

- If you had an abnormal Pap in the past
- If you've ever had a bacterial infection or sexually transmitted disease
- If you're currently sexually active
- If you have any symptoms of vaginitis
- If you suspect that you might be at risk for an STD
- If you have a history of cervical cancer in your family

Questions to Ask Your Doctor

- Is it ASC-US or ASC-H?
- Should I have an HPV test?
- Might the ASCUS on my Pap smear be due to anything other than HPV, such as vaginitis?
- Will I have colposcopy? If not, when will I come back for a follow-up Pap smear?
- Does my partner need to be examined?

CHAPTER FIVE

Abnormal Paps:
An LSIL Diagnosis

You have an abnormal Pap smear. Not just that, but your doctor says you have dysplasia or CIN (cervical intraepithelial neoplasia).

"I didn't think anything was really wrong with me, and then my doctor said, 'You have dysplasia, a precancerous condition caused by HPV,'" says Andrea, age thirty-four. "All I heard were 'cancer,' 'H,' and 'V.' I thought I was going to die."

The bad news is, dysplasia *is* a precancerous condition that, left untreated, could eventually lead to cancer. In addition, it's caused by HPV, so having an experience like Andrea's—hearing about cancer *and* an STD in one blow—can be traumatic.

Here's the good news: Although it's considered a "precancerous" condition, you should pay more attention to the "pre" than the "cancer." In fact, only a small percentage of dysplasia progresses to cancer, and almost all cases can be caught and treated before they have the chance to do that . . . *if* you're getting your regular Pap smears. And as we know from your HPV 101 class, with due vigilance, HPV should never lead to anything more than an abnormal Pap in the future.

What Is Dysplasia?

Let's look at the chart from chapter 1 again:

Class System Rating (Pap Smears)	Bethesda System Rating (Pap Smears)	Dysplasia System Rating (Tissue Biopsies)	CIN (Cervical Intraepithelial Neoplasia) System Rating (Tissue Biopsies)	HPV Relationship Rating
0	Unsatisfactory	Unsatisfactory	Unsatisfactory	Not enough evidence to say
1	Within normal limits	Negative	Negative	—
1	Benign cellular changes	Negative	Negative	—
2	ASC-US[1] or AGUS[2] favor reactive	No term	No term	+/−
2	ASC-H[3] or AGUS favor neoplasia	No term	No term	+/−
3	LSIL[4]	Mild	CIN 1	+
3	HSIL[5]	Moderate	CIN 2	+

Class System Rating (Pap Smears)	Bethesda System Rating (Pap Smears)	Dysplasia System Rating (Tissue Biopsies)	CIN (Cervical Intraepithelial Neoplasia) System Rating (Tissue Biopsies)	HPV Relationship Rating
3	HSIL	Severe	CIN 3	+
4	HSIL	CIS (carcinoma in situ)	CIN 3	+
5	Carcinoma	Carcinoma	Carcinoma	+

[1]AS-CUS = atypical squamous cells of undetermined significance
[2]AGUS = atypical glandular cells of undetermined significance
[3]ASC-H = atypical squamous cells; cannot exclude HSIL
[4]LSIL = low-grade squamous intraepithelial lesions
[5]HSIL = high-grade squamous intraepithelial lesions

That Awful Terminology!

We covered ASCUS in the last chapter, and we've already covered the description of what LSIL and HSIL look like under the microscope. To remind you, the class system and Bethesda system are used for Pap smears. The dysplasia system and CIN system are used to describe tissue samples. The term *LSIL*, used in the Bethesda system, stands for "low-grade squamous intraepithelial lesions." *Low-grade* is self-explanatory: The cellular changes are relatively mild. We know *squamous* describes the cells on the topmost layer of your cervix; *intraepithelial* means that all of the changes are above the basement membrane, i.e., still within the skin layer. Once cells cross the basement membrane and enter the tissues below, you have cancer.

The word *dysplasia* is another word for "intraepithelial

lesions" (see chart pages 116–17). The equivalent of LSIL is mild dysplasia or CIN 1, and the equivalent of HSIL is moderate (CIN 2) or severe (CIN 3) dysplasia.

The most advanced form of dysplasia is called *carcinoma in situ*. This is basically equivalent to severe dysplasia. Every now and then I have a clearly worried patient come into my office and tell me that she was told by her primary-care doctor that she has cancer. A perfectly good reason to be concerned! The problem is that when I do a little more digging, I find out that her biopsy showed carcinoma in situ, not cancer. The problem lies in the "carcinoma" part of the carcinoma in situ. The word *carcinoma* does mean cancer, but the "in situ" part means that it is still above the basement membrane—it isn't cancer at all!

Some doctors don't understand the difference between carcinoma in situ and true cancer, while many others do and, for some reason, don't explain that difference clearly enough to the patient. Problematic as it is, this sort of situation does provide me with a somewhat pleasant opportunity to instantly "cure" the patient of cancer. Of course, she remains in serious need of having the lesion removed to prevent cancer from developing. Like any other form of dysplasia, carcinoma in situ is still precancerous and is treated with local removal, while cancer often needs to be treated by means such as radiation or chemotherapy.

Even though LSIL is a more serious condition than ASCUS, most doctors—myself included—recommend a follow-up Pap smear every three to six months, since more than half of LSIL diagnoses spontaneously regress. If the next series of Pap smears are normal, then you can return to the usual schedule of annual Pap smear testing. On the other hand, if any of the follow-up Pap smears is abnormal, then most doctors would recommend colposcopy for further evaluation.

Some doctors perform colposcopy at the first sign of LSIL on a Pap smear. Why, when I already said LSIL doesn't lead to cancer? The answer is that about 25 percent of women with LSIL on a Pap smear will have moderate or severe dysplasia at colposcopy. Remember, the Pap smear grading system isn't meant to indicate the true severity of a cervical lesion—ASCUS on a Pap smear can indicate anything from mild dysplasia to severe dysplasia. The Pap smear is primarily used to identify who needs further evaluation, while the severity is determined on a tissue biopsy.

A few other LSIL situations should trigger an immediate colposcopy. If I'm concerned that you may not return for regular follow-up visits, I strongly consider colposcopy and treatment of the lesion as soon as possible. If you're known to be immunosuppressed for any reason, including HIV infection, I perform colposcopy. Finally, if you request it, I perform colposcopy.

As far as your general health goes, if your LSIL result on the Pap corresponds to a mild diagnosis on a biopsy, this isn't a serious condition. The seriousness of mild dysplasia comes with what it *indicates*: the presence of HPV. At this point, the presence of HPV is definite, and although the lesions may regress, as I said in chapter 1, it's possible that the virus may *not* go away. Remember, too, that mild dysplasia is considered to be the most infectious stage of HPV infection.

Even more important, mild dysplasia has the potential to progress to moderate or severe (about 15 to 20 percent will progress), which, in turn, can progress to cancer. Most doctors believe mild dysplasia doesn't progress directly to cancer, so it's not precancerous by itself. Remember, though, that most mild dysplasia contains cancer-causing HPV types, so it can be considered *indirectly* precancerous. Bear in mind, though, that most mild dysplasia won't progress to a higher grade of disease.

Although most mild dysplasias are associated with oncogenic HPV types, some are associated with low-risk types such as HPV 6 or 11. If you've been infected with 6 or 11, you may develop bumpy, cauliflower-like warts on the surface of your cervix. You may or may not also find warts on your vulva or vagina. In fact, warts are considered to be a form of mild dysplasia. These warts won't lead to cancer, but keep in mind that having 6 or 11 doesn't rule out the possibility of carrying one of the cancer-causing types, too.

In fact, like other sexually transmitted agents, HPVs like to travel in packs. If you're at risk for one HPV type, you're at risk for other HPV types as well. Some people have two or more HPV types at once, and women who have warts on their vulva or vagina are at higher risk of having dysplasia than women without warts—even if their external warts and cervical disease are caused by different HPV types. I'll cover genital warts and their treatment in chapters 11 and 12.

Symptoms of LSIL

Patients are usually shocked to hear they have LSIL on a Pap smear. "But I'm *fine*," they say. You're probably used to illnesses with outward symptoms, like the itching of a yeast infection, the burning of a urinary tract infection, or even the lump in the breast that could signal breast cancer.

Unfortunately, the very reason that HPV infection is so common and so dangerous, the reason why so many women have it and so few have even heard of it, is that HPV is often a subclinical infection. *It shows no outward symptoms.* In fact, for most of you, you may only become aware of cervical HPV infection when you find out your Pap smear is abnormal. If you wait and develop symptoms of invasive cervical cancer such as bleeding and cramping, it could already have spread to nearby organs, such as your ovaries or uterus, and the damage may be irreversible.

On the other hand, as I said earlier, warts are a form of low-grade disease, and if these are present on your outer genitalia, they may cause symptoms such as burning, itching, and bleeding.

Dysplasia usually exhibits no outward symptoms. However, the changes of dysplasia are *completely reversible.* Those early stages can only be identified through a Pap smear. *Regular Pap smears save lives.*

Treatment of Mild Dysplasia

In most situations, most doctors—myself included—don't recommend treatment for mild dysplasia. This stage often regresses to normal, and advanced procedures are unnecessary. But if the mild progresses to moderate or severe dysplasia, your doctor should remove the tissue immediately.

Occasionally, treating mild dysplasia is a good idea. The treatment is the same as for moderate or severe dysplasia, and the treatment methods are described in more detail in chapter 6. If the dysplasia is persistent on follow-up, and shows no signs of regressing over time, talk to your doctor about treatment. Sometimes, mild cases are worth treating—even without follow-up—if it isn't clear that you'll return for all of your follow-up visits. If you can't assure adequate follow-up, then the prudent course would be to treat the mild dysplasia rather than risk progressing to untreated moderate or severe dysplasia. And of course, if you have warts, you'll probably want to have those treated, and this is discussed in chapter 12.

Pregnancy and Mild Dysplasia

As with ASCUS, a wait-and-see approach is usually the best for both pregnant and nonpregnant women with mild dysplasia. Since pregnancy lowers your immunity, it may increase your chance of advancing to moderate or severe dysplasia. Another consideration is HPV reactivation. Discuss the consequences with your doctor: Could you possibly pass HPV on to your child? HPV can be passed on to infants during a vaginal delivery, increasing your child's chance of developing papillomatosis in his or her esophagus, lungs, or larynx. (These conditions are discussed in chapter 13.) Rarely, large cervical warts could block the exit for the baby. In these very unusual cases, a cesarean section may be necessary.

Immunosuppression and Dysplasia

Traditionally, the most common form of immunosuppression in women was that associated with organ transplants, especially kidneys. To prevent rejection of the new organ by the body, doctors give medicines to suppress the immune system. Unfortunately, that affects the whole immune system, including immunity to viruses such as HPV. Consequently, women with kidney transplants are at increased risk of cervical HPV infection, dysplasia, and cervical cancer. They're also at increased risk of vaginal and vulvar cancers.

More recently, human immunodeficiency virus (HIV) has emerged as the most common cause of immunosuppression. There is a large body of literature that shows that, like the women with transplants, HIV-positive women are at increased risk for cervical HPV infection, dysplasia, and cervical cancer. HIV-positive women tend to have more HPV types in their cervix and vagina than do HIV-negative women, and they tend to progress faster to moderate or severe stages. In general, the more advanced the HIV disease is, the higher the risk of dysplasia. There is also more difficulty in treating moderate or severe cases, and sometimes several different treatment approaches are needed.

Similarly, if an HIV-positive woman develops cervical cancer, treating the cancer can be much more difficult than in an otherwise healthy woman. As I indicated earlier, HIV-positive women are advised to have a comprehensive gynecologic examination and a Pap smear as part of their initial medical evaluation. If initial results are normal, at least one additional Pap should be obtained six months later to exclude a false-negative result on the initial smear. If the second smear is normal, HIV-infected women could have annual smears, similar to HIV-negative women. If the initial or follow-up cytology shows ASCUS or SIL, the woman should be referred for a colposcopy.

How Can I Prevent Future Mild Dysplasia?

Although HPV infection is not curable at present, improving and maintaining your general health can help prevent future abnormal Pap smears and dysplasia. Makes sense, right? Healthy lives lead to healthy bodies. Many factors contribute to the leap from HPV infection to dysplasia, and I've included a list of risk factors below. Some of them—such as HPV infection itself, sex before the age of seventeen, and family history—are unchangeable. But you could help to stack the odds more in your favor if you keep up your health in other areas and make sure they're the only risk factors.

The risk factors for dysplasia are the same for cervical cancer, and keep in mind that because HPV is a risk factor, all factors for HPV (outlined in chapter 1) also apply here.

Risk Factors for Dysplasia

- **HPV infection.** If you have HPV, you have the one factor that is *necessary* for dysplasia, and therefore cancer, to develop.
- **History of STDs.** Any infection and subsequent treatment can weaken the cervix and make it vulnerable to cellular changes. Although your current history cannot be changed, more communication with your sexual partners and using condoms can prevent future STDs.
- **Smoking.** Smoking weakens your immune system. It fills your body with carcinogens and accelerates the degeneration of normal cells into abnormal cells. *Smoking kills.*
- **Stress.** There is some suggestion that psychological stress may weaken your immune system. Do what you can to lower the stress level in your life.

- **Family history.** If your family has a history of cervical cancer, your chances of developing dysplasia (and thus cancer) may be increased. Lucky for you, though, you know what the risk factors are and can stop the development early on.
- **Poor nutrition and/or obesity.** Some studies have shown that a balanced diet of folic acid and vitamins C and E can increase your cervix's ability to fight off the HPV infection. Eat your fruits and vegetables!
- **Oral contraceptive use.** The relationship between birth control pills and cervical cancer has been heavily debated. One reason could be that fewer women who use oral contraceptives use condoms, thus increasing their chances of transmitting HPV. Another reason is that the steroids in the pill may stimulate HPV proteins. In either case, the effect is likely to be weak.
- **Age.** Although women under age thirty are more likely to have HPV infection, cervical cancer and severe dysplasia are far more common in women thirty years or older. Loss of immunity and menopause could contribute to this increased incidence, so older women are especially reminded to get Pap smears.
- **HIV, pregnancy, and other immunity-compromised conditions.** As with poor nutrition, decreased immunity means increased risk. Many HIV-positive patients, pregnant women, and recent recipients of organ transplants experience dysplasia because their bodies aren't as capable of keeping HPV in check.
- **Low socioeconomic status.** Although poor general health contributes to a decrease in immunity, poor *health care*—meaning lack of insurance, money, and regular doctor visits—increases your risk of advancing beyond dysplasia to cervical cancer. Women with less money and access to health care are less likely to get Paps and are therefore less likely to find cancer in its early stages. In developing countries, cervical cancer is the most common killer of women simply because they don't have the means to get regular Paps.

A combination of any or all of these factors can contribute to your chance of developing dysplasia and/or cervical cancer, but the one *necessary* element is HPV infection. Knowing that you have HPV and that your great-aunt and grandmother died of cervical cancer actually puts you at an advantage: You *know* you're at high risk. So you *know* that you need to quit smoking, eat a balanced diet, keep your stress levels to a minimum, choose your sexual partners wisely, and get annual Pap smears. Once you do all of those things, you're once again in control of your sexual health. Again I want to stress one important point: Eating well, not smoking, and lowering your stress level are all critical to healthy living and they may well contribute to regression of dysplasia. On the other hand, dysplasia may persist or progress in even the healthiest of women. The message? Do everything you can to remain healthy, but if your dysplasia does not go away by itself, it's almost certainly not your fault!

A Word on Nutrition

A healthy lifestyle often starts with a healthy diet, and many studies have been conducted about the effect of diet on abnormal Pap smears and dysplasia. The research is still in its early stages, but some results have shown that women with folic acid and vitamin deficiencies (often anorexic or bulimic women) have higher rates of dysplasia. A diet rich in fruits and vegetables, including retinoids and vitamins C and E, may increase your immunity and your ability to keep HPV infection under control. Several studies have shown that antioxidants have been found to decrease the chance of developing dysplasia, and since *you're* the only one in control of your diet, you may be able to help prevent future dysplasia.

Antioxidants are most abundant in fruits, fruit juices, green, leafy vegetables, and orange and red vegetables. Supplements may help if you're unable or unwilling to take in the daily recommendations in government guidelines (remember the food pyramid?). The recommended daily allowance (RDA) for folic acid is 400 micrograms, 60 milligrams for vitamin C, and 30 International Units (IUs) for vitamin E. I recommend taking up to 500 milligrams of vitamin C and 100 IUs of vitamin E, since the RDA may fall below what your body needs. Most multivitamins include 100 percent of the RDA, and for the extra boost, just about any drugstore sells vitamins C and E these days.

Although taking vitamin supplements won't guarantee protection against dysplasia, it certainly couldn't hurt. Keep in mind, though, that as is the case with just about anything in life, more isn't always better. Taking excessive vitamins can lead to serious side effects. Too much vitamin A can lead to problems in the brain, and vitamin E is not recommended for anyone taking anticoagulant drugs.

Conclusion

Although finding out you have a sexually transmitted disease is traumatic, take heart! When properly followed or treated, mild dysplasia shouldn't lead to serious problems. Mild cases often regress to normal; even if they advance to moderate or severe, treatments are available to remove the affected area. Maintaining your health through not smoking, eating well, controlling your mental stress level, staying physically fit, and getting regular Pap smears could keep HPV infection from ever advancing beyond this stage. Staying healthy is critical, but despite all of your best efforts, dysplastic cells may still go their merry ways. Don't blame yourself if it doesn't go away by itself.

Topics to Discuss with Your Doctor

Tell Your Doctor . . .

- If you had an abnormal Pap in the past
- If you ever had a sexually transmitted disease
- If you are currently sexually active
- If you have a history of cervical cancer in your family

Questions to Ask Your Doctor

- Will I have a colposcopy?
- If not, when will I come back for a follow-up Pap smear?
- Should I change any of my personal habits to prevent this from happening again?
- What should I tell my partner?
- Does my partner need to be examined?
- What other developments should I expect?

CHAPTER SIX

Abnormal Paps:
An HSIL Diagnosis

Perhaps you've already had several abnormal Pap smears. Maybe you had ASCUS and your doctor advised you to come back in three months. Perhaps a diagnosis of HSIL (high-grade squamous intraepithelial lesion) on the Pap smear was your first clue that anything might be wrong in your cervix. In any case, HSIL on a Pap smear is serious and requires further diagnostic procedures and treatment. (Figure 2.2 shows a Pap smear with HSIL.)

Why? When your Pap smear shows evidence of HSIL, a colposcopy and biopsy will probably confirm moderate or severe dysplasia in the cervix. Remember, LSIL on a Pap *could* mean moderate or severe dysplasia on the cervix, but HSIL on a Pap smear *usually* means that. That said, these stages are not life-threatening—as long as you get treatment and return for all of your follow-up Pap smears. Figure 2.3 shows the appearance of the cervix with severe dysplasia and figure 2.4 shows a microscopic view of a severe dysplasia biopsy.

I know it sounds complicated. But just look at it this way: If someone tells you it's hot outside, you know you need to wear shorts and sandals as opposed to jeans and boots. A meteorologist, though, will consider all the factors of the heat: Is it 85 or 105 degrees? Is it incredibly humid? Has it been hot for a long time? Is a low-pressure system coming in? Is a cold front moving in? If it's 85 and sunny, then you just want to make sure you wear suntan lotion. If, on the other hand, it's overcast, 105, humid, the barometer's dropping, and a cold front's rushing in, then you might want to buy some emergency candles and brace yourself for a heck of a thunderstorm. In the case of dysplasia, the Pap smear just says, "It's hot." Your doctor knows to check all the other factors and signs—through colposcopy—to make sure you aren't headed for a storm of your own.

What Are Moderate and Severe Dysplasia?

Moderate and severe dysplasia, but *especially* severe dysplasia, are the next-to-last step in the progression of cell abnormalities, with invasive cancer being the last step. It's your last chance to stop cervical cancer in its tracks! However, as I've been implying, the risk of progressing to cancer from moderate dysplasia is probably not as high as the risk of progressing to cancer from severe dysplasia. Without treatment, moderate and severe dysplasia may advance to invasive cancer within an unpredictable number of years, *unpredictable* meaning there's no way of knowing how long it will take—ten months or ten years (usually years).

To remind you, moderate and severe dysplasia are characterized by the replacement of most of the normal cervical cells with cells that can become cancerous, but no one knows for sure what makes that happen. Several changes occur in these cells that could make them cancerous. First, HPV has slowed down or stopped making viral particles. It's not really trying to infect any more cells at this point. Second, more and more of the proteins that cause cancerous changes are being made in the bottom layers of the cervix. (Remember, in mild dysplasia, these proteins are usually found in the mature, higher layers of the cervix.) As I explained in chapter 1, it seems likely, though, that these proteins contribute to the accumulation of more and more genetic damage, which in turn contributes to the malignancy and an inability of the cells to stop dividing. That's when the real danger for invasive cancer begins: when cancer cells divide beyond your body's ability to stop them and could potentially spread deeper into your tissue.

Although these cases can develop gradually, after a series of ASCUS or LSIL Paps, many women develop moderate or severe dysplasia without ever having any previous indication of HPV infection or signs of HPV-associated cervical disease. In one study of college-age women, moderate or severe dysplasia developed within an average of two years from the time of initial HPV infection. It's likely that development of dysplasia takes even longer than that in many women.

The rate of progress to moderate or severe dysplasia

depends on several viral and environmental factors. Although moderate or severe dysplasia nearly always indicates the presence of a high-risk HPV type, not all cancer-causing types are alike in their risk. Remember that in chapter 1, I said that not all versions of a given HPV type are alike. Multiple versions exist of a given HPV type, such as HPV 16, and these are called *variants.* For example, some HPV 16 variants are more aggressive than others. So if you're unlucky enough to have one of the more aggressive variants of a cancer-causing HPV type, it's possible that your risk of developing moderate or severe dysplasia is higher, or it may develop more quickly. In addition, smoking affects your immune response to the virus, and tobacco smoke contains several cancer-causing compounds. Those compounds may cause DNA damage in cells, especially if the cells can't repair the damage when they're infected with HPV, because of the E6 protein. Remember, the E6 protein leads to the destruction of your p53 protein, one of the cellular proteins that helps repair DNA damage in a cell. Genetic predisposition probably plays a role by determining your immune response as well.

Let's look at the chart again.

Abnormal Class	Regression to Normal	Progression to Higher Grade over 24 months	Progression to Invasive Cancer over 24 months
ASCUS	68%	7%	0.25%
LSIL	47%	21%	0.15%
HSIL	35%	23%	1.44%

HSIL on a Pap smear has half the chance of ASCUS for regression, and is over three times more likely to advance to a higher grade of lesion, which is why further diagnosis and treatment are necessary. At this point, your doctor will recommend a colposcopy. Once the diagnosis of moderate or severe dysplasia is confirmed in the tissue sample (biopsy) and cancer is ruled out, you'll need treatment.

Treatment of Moderate or Severe Dysplasia

After your doctor receives the results of the biopsy—which will indicate the severity of your dysplasia, and the best treatment option—he or she will probably ask you to come to the office for one of several procedures: Loop electrosurgical excision procedure (LEEP), conization, or cryotherapy. Unfortunately, we really don't have any methods to treat HPV itself. (We're all hoping this will change, and some of the more promising new approaches are described in chapter 16.) So for the moment, we're stuck with methods that seem pretty archaic—physical removal or destruction of the diseased tissue. Since these methods don't treat HPV per se, some HPV infection may be left behind, perhaps in a few spots in the normal-looking tissue remaining after the treatment. This remaining HPV has the potential to reactivate and cause a recurrence of the lesion.

The Loop Electrosurgical Excision Procedure (LEEP)

The loop electrosurgical excision procedure (LEEP) is the most commonly used procedure for removal of moderate or severe dysplasia. (Another term for the procedure is *LLETZ*, large loop excision of the transformation zone.) In fact, LEEP is used to both diagnose and treat dysplasia. Using a thin wire loop electrode (see fig. 2.6) attached to an electrical generator, an electrical current quickly cuts away cervical tissue in the immediate area of the loop wire. The procedure is performed in your doctor's office and is quick. Depending on whether anesthesia is used, it's usually relatively painless.

Again, you'll have your feet in the stirrups and a speculum in place, and your doctor will use a colposcope to view the procedure. Your doctor will place an electrosurgical dispersive pad (a gel-covered adhesive electrode) on your thigh to provide a safe return path for the electric current. He or she will then attach a disposable loop electrode to the generator hand-piece and apply vinegar to look for acetowhitening.

At this point, you'll either be given a local or, more rarely, a general anesthetic. With a local, you'll remain awake during the procedure, while a general anesthetic will put you to sleep (in either case, you should bring a friend along to drive you home). In addition, you may want to take ibuprofen beforehand to minimize any pain following the procedure. Don't take aspirin, also known as acetylsalicylic acid (ASA), though; it thins your blood and could increase bleeding.

After the anesthesia takes effect, your doctor will pass the wire loop through the surface of your cervix. After the lesion is removed, he or she will use an electrode to stop any bleeding, and may apply a solution to the remaining tissue to prevent further bleeding.

Your doctor will send the removed tissue to the lab to provide a more accurate assessment of the abnormal area, as well as to make sure that the entire lesion was removed. To determine if the entire lesion was removed, the pathologist looks at the outer edges of the tissue. If any signs of dysplasia show at the edges of the removed tissue, the pathologist calls this a "positive margin." This means there's a high likelihood that some dysplasia remains in the cervix after the LEEP. If this is the case, then you'll need to be reassessed for persistent dysplasia and possibly re-treated.

After your LEEP, you may experience mild pain, similar to menstrual cramps, and light bleeding. If the pain feels excessive, the bleeding is more than a normal period, or you experience heavy vaginal discharge or strong odor, call your doctor.

Recovery from LEEP usually lasts about three weeks, and during this time, you should not have sexual intercourse, lift heavy objects, use tampons, or douche. Any of the above activities could cause increased bleeding, pain, and a longer healing time.

You'll usually be examined within a few weeks of your LEEP to make sure that you're healing well and showing no signs of cervical stenosis (scarring leading to blocking of menstrual blood flow from the uterus). You'll probably be asked to return for follow-up Paps every three months for a year, then every six months until your doctor decides you can return to a yearly exam. You *must* return for your follow-up Paps: Your doctor has to make sure you've healed properly, that the entire abnormal area was removed, and that no new abnormalities have developed.

Although LEEP does remove the entire affected area and all abnormal cells, *it does not remove the HPV virus.* To say that the only site of HPV infection is where the dysplasia was detected and treated is risky at best. HPV may remain dormant in or around the cervix even after any procedure. HPV can also hang out in the vagina, vulva, or anus.

LEEP is the treatment of choice for several reasons. First, this procedure preserves the margins of the excised tissue very well, so the pathologist can assess it more accurately. Occasionally LEEP singes the outside edges of the biopsy, possible masking more serious abnormalities, and in that case, a surgical cone biopsy (dicussed next) may be necessary.

Second, it's associated with fewer side effects than other treatment methods. The development of side effects is related to the amount of tissue removed and may include bleeding during or after the procedure. Rare side effects include cervical stenosis or cervical incompetence, a cervix too weak to hold the baby in, which can lead to preterm delivery and low birth weight.

Third, it's usually effective in treating the lesion. Most or all of the transformation zone is removed in the procedure, and as you recall, the transformation zone is the favorite area for HPV to infect and cause a lesion. If you remove that vulnerable tissue, then the risk of a recurrent lesion is very small. One of the disadvantages of LEEP is its cost— it's relatively expensive when compared to procedures commonly used in the past, such as cryosurgery, described later in this chapter.

Cone Biopsy or Conization

The cone biopsy, like LEEP, can be both a diagnostic procedure and treatment for dysplasia. A diagram showing this procedure is shown in figure 6.1. The procedure is also known as "cold-knife" conization. Instead of using the electrical loop, the tissue is removed with a surgical scalpel. Using the scalpel, your doctor removes a cone-shaped sample of the affected tissue for further study. The procedure is usually done in an ambulatory surgery setting (also known as day surgery) as opposed to a doctor's office, and is usually done under general anesthesia. Cone biopsies are performed instead of LEEP when your doctor is more concerned about cervical cancer, if the colposcopy was unsatisfactory, or if the endocervical curettage was positive, indicating the possibility of serious cervical disease that can't be directly seen by the doctor.

Cone biopsies are typically performed only if the patient cannot be treated with LEEP or laser conization (discussed later) and is associated with a higher complication rate than the other procedures, including bleeding, stenosis, and scarring. Some of the complications of surgical cone biopsies are related to having general anesthesia.

After conization, you may experience some bleeding and cramping for a few days; any excessive bleeding or pain should be immediately reported to your doctor. You may want to restrict any heavy activity, like cardiovascular workouts, for two weeks, and you should not have sex, use tampons, or douche for at least four weeks. As with the LEEP, you will usually be examined within a few weeks of your procedure to make sure that you are healing well and that

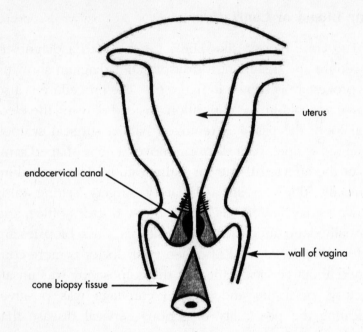

Figure 6.1: A Cone Biopsy. *In a cone biopsy, a cone-shaped portion of the cervix containing the transformation zone is removed. If the lesion extends into the endocervical canal, a larger proportion of the endocervical canal is removed with a longer cone. (Illustration reprinted by permission of Mosby-Year Books, Inc., St. Louis, Missouri, 64146. Photo originally appeared in DiSaia and Creasman,* Clinical Gynecologic Oncology, *Fifth edition, 1997.)*

there are no signs of cervical stenosis developing. Again, always return for your follow-up Pap smear in three months.

Cryotherapy

Cryotherapy, or freezing, was used often in the past, but it's used less and less these days. It's a simple procedure—your doctor places a probe (cooled to an extremely low temperature by liquid nitrogen) against your cervix. This cools the entire cervix to subzero temperatures, effectively creating a temporary cervical ice ball. The probe is typically applied twice for two to three minutes at a time and leads to destruction of the frozen areas. While it uses inexpensive equipment and can be performed in an office setting, its primary disadvantage is a high failure rate for treating large areas of dysplasia.

For about a month after freezing, the cells damaged by freezing shed in a heavy watery discharge. When the cervix heals, usually within two to three months, scarring may occur. This may make it harder to interpret future Pap smears and colposcopies. Later Pap smears are often unsatisfactory and the scars may hide new lesions. Finally, cryotherapy is not suitable for women with unsatisfactory colposcopy, a positive ECC, or especially large lesions.

As a rule, cryotherapy is most effective in treating mild dysplasia, and since most mild dysplasia doesn't require treatment, other methods of excision are preferable.

Laser Conization

Laser conization with a carbon dioxide (CO_2) laser is another treatment approach. Performed with the help of the colposcope, it allows the doctor to control the depth of the lesion excision and minimize damage to surrounding tissues. The laser seals blood vessels, so the risk of bleeding is lower than with some other therapies. Healing typically occurs without the scarring associated with cryosurgery, creating more accurate follow-up cytology and colposcopy.

Laser therapy is usually performed in an office setting with local anesthesia. Like cryotherapy, it shouldn't be used for women with unsatisfactory colposcopy, a positive ECC, or especially large lesions. With the advent of LEEP, the popularity of laser has waned.

Other Procedures: Hysterectomy and Topical Therapies

Hysterectomy (the surgical removal of the uterus and cervix) can be performed if fertility is not a factor and if other gynecologic indications are present, such as bleeding or pain from fibroids of the uterus. It should rarely, if ever, be used if the *only* indication is moderate or severe dysplasia. Topical therapies such as retinoic acid and 5-fluorouracil (Efudex) have not been shown to be adequate as primary treatment of moderate or severe dysplasia.

Fertility and Moderate or Severe Dysplasia

Your cervix needs time to heal and rebuild after a surgical procedure. A cone biopsy or cryotherapy could lead to cervical stenosis, scarring, or cervical incompetence. These complications are very rare, but if it's been a year since your procedure and you still haven't conceived in the traditional way, you may want to see a fertility specialist about further workup and possibly consider other avenues such as artificial insemination.

If you're trying to get pregnant now and your Pap comes back abnormal, you, your partner, and your doctor can decide together what your options are. Dysplasia itself won't cause infertility. If your Pap shows ASCUS or LSIL, you probably won't need any procedures, anyway. Keep in mind, though, that pregnancy does impair your immune system, so be vigilant about watching the progress of your Pap.

Pregnancy and Moderate or Severe Dysplasia

Treatment of prenatal moderate or severe dysplasia has been the subject of debate: Wait and see? Treat immediately? Most doctors recommend a colposcopy, as this doesn't harm the fetus in any way. In general, doctors try to disturb the cervix as little as possible during pregnancy. However, if colposcopy reveals a suspicious lesion, a biopsy may be necessary to rule out the possibility of moderate or severe dysplasia or invasive cancer.

Once you know your diagnosis is moderate or severe, you can discuss your options with your doctor. Conization has been shown to increase the chance of premature delivery (El-Bastawissi et al. 1999), and cryotherapy is rarely recommended in this situation.

Often, though, the best route is to defer treatment until after you've given birth. The presence of moderate or severe dysplasia could increase your baby's chances of acquiring HPV during a vaginal birth, but even so, doctors wouldn't recommend a cesarean section for this reason. Since pregnancy only lasts nine months, the possibility of moderate or severe dysplasia advancing to cervical cancer is slim. If you do develop cervical cancer, then it's still best to wait until late in the pregnancy to begin any cancer treatment, but the baby should be delivered as early as possible.

Of course, returning for follow-up treatments is necessary immediately after you've had your baby. As we discussed earlier, some cases of moderate or severe dysplasia may even regress on their own after delivery. Though you can defer treatment of moderate or severe dysplasia, the sooner it's treated, the better—and the sooner you can enjoy being a mother without the specter of cervical cancer hanging over your head.

Preventing Future Moderate and Severe Dysplasia

The recurrence rate after LEEP and conization are low; usually these procedures remove all affected cells, and if the follow-up Pap smears are normal, they'll probably stay normal unless some outside factor is introduced. For instance, many women who have had normal Paps for years redevelop dysplasia when they become pregnant, acquire HIV, or suffer a similar condition that suppresses the immune system. If the follow-up Pap shows abnormal cells, then the severity of the lesion (determined during colposcopy and biopsy) will determine whether you need to repeat the treatment.

In general, in the year after a removal procedure, you should have follow-up Paps every three months. If you're still in the clear after twelve months, every six months should suffice until your doctor feels comfortable with annual Paps.

The best ways to avoid future bouts of dysplasia are outlined in chapter 5. Good health and nutrition are important for boosting your immunity, so do your best to quit smoking and start eating your fruits and vegetables today! These may not be enough, however, so it's also critical that you return for all of your follow-up visits.

Dysplasia and Your Partner

Because dysplasia indicates the presence of HPV, you do need to discuss the infection with your current and previous partners, whether they may have infected you or vice versa. If you've had several recent partners, there's no practical way to find out who gave it to you, but the three-to-four-month incubation period is a fairly good indication of initial infection. Keep in mind, though, that HPV infections can remain latent for months or years.

Because of the silent, subclinical nature of HPV, your partner may assume "it isn't him." Let him know that HPV does not show up in a blood test, nor is an HPV DNA test available for testing the penis only. All you can do at this point is let him know the risks for infecting future partners. (The effect of oncogenic HPV on men is covered more thoroughly in chapters 14 and 15.)

As for broaching the subject with future partners, refer to chapter 15, "Living with HPV and Talking with Your Partner."

Conclusion

Whether your doctor calls it moderate or severe dysplasia, carcinoma in situ, CIN 2, CIN 3 or HSIL, this stage is critical in the development of cancer. With treatment, it can be eradicated. Without treatment, you could develop cervical cancer in a few years or a few months. Your Pap smear indicates only that you have a serious condition, so further diagnostic procedures such as colposcopy and biopsy are essential to judge the level of the lesion.

As I've mentioned in previous chapters, because you know your diagnosis, you're at an advantage. You *know* you're at risk for cervical cancer. After your LEEP or conization, you can change your lifestyle to lessen your risk for developing dysplasia again—eat well, reduce the stress in your life, and if possible, quit smoking. Even with these important measures, however, the dysplasia can still come back. Now that you know from experience that a Pap smear potentially saved your life, you'll go to your doctor for follow-up Pap smears to confirm that you're still in the clear. If you do develop abnormalities in the future, you know how to deal with them.

Questions to Ask Your Doctor

- Do I have moderate dysplasia or severe dysplasia?
- When should I come in for my colposcopy?
- What kind of treatment procedure will I have?
- What is the advantage of this treatment over the other available treatments?

- What is the success rate of your recommended treatment?
- Should I take ibuprofen or some other painkiller before my colposcopy/LEEP/conization/cryotherapy?
- Which drugs should I not take before a procedure, like aspirin?
- Should I bring a friend with me for my LEEP/conization/cryotherapy?
- Will I experience any side effects?
- What should I do to lessen the side effects of my procedure?
- Was all of the dysplastic tissue removed?
- When should I come in for my follow-up Pap smear?
- How often after my initial follow-up should I come in?
- What can I do to prevent future dysplasia?
- What should I tell my partner?
- Does my partner need to be examined?

CHAPTER SEVEN

Cervical Cancer

Before the invention of the Pap smear in the 1940s, cervical cancer was the most deadly cancer for women in the United States. Since regular screenings began, that rate has dropped nearly 77 percent among Caucasian women, but it still remains the second most common cancer in the world, and the most common in some developing countries.

Cervical Cancer Stats

A disproportionate number of women with cervical cancer belong to a minority group. In general, cervical cancer strikes women of lower socioeconomic status. Why? Without proper screening and follow-up, cervical cancer can be fatal, and women with little or no access to medical care can't afford or don't have access to Pap smear screening and other diagnostic procedures. In addition, the mortality rate among African-American women remains higher than among Caucasian women, even after treatment.

The survival rate of cervical cancer depends on the stage; in the early stages (Stage II-A or less), there's a good to excellent five-year survival rate, but women with more advanced tumors tend to do poorly. However, recent developments using a combination of chemotherapy and radiation therapy have shown excellent long-term results for advanced-stage cancers.

What Is Cervical Cancer?

As frightening as the word *cancer* can be, few people know what it actually *is.* Up to the point of severe dysplasia, the abnormal cells are still on top of the basement membrane and have not invaded below. Cancer occurs when your body's most basic unit, the cell, becomes abnormal, invades the basement membrane, and divides without control or order (see fig. 1.3). The abnormal cells then invade deeper and deeper into surrounding tissues and may spread to distant parts of the body as well.

When new cells are not needed but are still uncontrollably produced, they create a mass of extra tissue: a tumor. Genital warts are considered to be benign tumors, meaning that they're not cancerous; polyps and cysts are other common benign growths of the cervix. These cells produce tumors that may grow large in some cases, but they don't spread to distant parts of the body or invade and destroy vital organs.

In contrast, *malignant* tumors may spread locally and block or destroy vital organs such as the uterus, bladder, or ovaries, or they may spread and sprout up in distant parts of the body, where other organs may be damaged or destroyed. The term for distant spread is *metastasis*. Metastasis typically occurs when the cells spread through the bloodstream, or via the lymph node system, to distant parts of the body. Although cervical cancer usually spreads locally and affects organs close to the cervix, cervical cancer cells can also break away and metastasize to organs like the lungs or liver.

Symptoms

As I stated in previous chapters, early stages of cervical cancer don't exhibit any outward symptoms. Once the cancer becomes invasive, the most common symptom is abnormal bleeding, which may occur between menstrual periods, after sex, douching, or a pelvic exam. Period bleeding may be heavier or last longer, and postmenopausal bleeding can also indicate cervical cancer. Increased vaginal discharge may also occur.

Pain is another sign of cervical cancer. If the tumor is advanced, it may invade nerves or block organs, causing pain. Another sign of cancer is swollen lymph nodes. If the cancer has spread to the groin (the term in medicalese is *inguinal*) lymph nodes, then a woman may note new swellings on one or both sides in her groin.

Diagnosis

As I've said a dozen times before, a Pap test is the most common, most effective screening technique to prevent cervical cancer. A technical point here: You'll often hear people say that the Pap smear's a screening test for cervical cancer. In reality, it isn't—it's really a screening test for dysplasia, because we want to detect and treat these lesions before they progress to cancer. So the Pap smear is really a screening test for *precancerous* lesions.

Having said that, on occasion, cervical cancer *is* diagnosed on a Pap smear, and our goal is to make this as rare as possible. In reality, the Pap smear is a lousy screening test for cervical cancer. Do you remember how I told you that the Pap test has only limited sensitivity for dysplasia? Well, it may be even worse for cervical cancer, and in a way this makes sense. Why? Many of the cancer cells that might otherwise be detectable on a Pap smear aren't found on the slide because they've invaded into the deep tissues. They're not accessible using a cytobrush—a brush designed to collect cells—or wooden spatula applied to the surface of the cervix in a routine Pap smear.

So sometimes, cervical cancer is diagnosed on a Pap smear. More often, though, the Pap smear shows LSIL or HSIL, and the *colposcopy* shows cervical cancer. Some of you may have read an article about HPV in *The New Yorker* (September, 1999) by Dr. Jerome Groopman. Yours truly was mentioned in it, and after the article came out, I was flooded with requests for more information about HPV and anogenital disease. In fact, the sheer volume of letters and messages that I received provided the major inspiration for me to write this book.

In that article, a patient who had a Pap smear result showing ASCUS was diagnosed within a short period of time with cervical cancer. The point of highlighting that patient was to illustrate that even relatively benign Pap smears might signal the presence of something far more serious, and that all abnormal Pap smears need to be taken seriously. Of course, I agree with that! However, as one of the individuals who provided information for that article, I also wanted to make clear that this situation is very unusual—if you look at a group of women with ASCUS on their Pap smear, only a very small proportion would be expected to have cervical cancer at that time, or even to develop it within a short time. So again, the message is, if you have an abnormal Pap smear, even with ASCUS, *don't* panic. *Do* have it followed up by your doctor.

To make a tissue diagnosis of cervical cancer, your physician may perform a colposcopy (described in chapter 4) or cone biopsy (described in chapter 6). Each of these procedures removes abnormal tissue and produces a biopsy, or sample. If the biopsy shows that a tumor exists or that the abnormal cells have invaded surrounding tissue, then a diagnosis of cervical cancer has been confirmed. At this point, you'll need to go through staging, a careful attempt to find out how much of your body has been affected by the cancer.

Staging of Cervical Cancer

Like the precancerous stages, mild through severe dysplasia, cervical cancer has been divided into several stages for descriptive and treatment purposes. Here's a chart to indicate the various stages.

Stage	What It Means
0	Also known as carcinoma in situ (a variant of severe dysplasia), the cells haven't invaded the deeper tissues of the cervix. Basically, this isn't really cancer.
I-A	A very small amount of cancer, visible only under a microscope, is found deeper in tissues of the cervix. The lesion is less than 5 mm deep, from the base of the epithelium from which it originates, and does not exceed 7 mm in horizontal spread.
I-B	A larger amount of cancer than in type I-A is found in the tissues of the cervix, but the tumor does not extend beyond the cervix.
II-A	Cancer has spread beyond the cervix to the upper two-thirds of the vagina.
II-B	Cancer has spread to the tissue around the cervix but not to the sidewalls of the pelvis.
III	Cancer has spread throughout the pelvic area, and cancer cells may have spread to the lower one-third of the vagina. The cells also may have spread to block the tubes connecting the kidney and bladder (the ureters).
IV-A	Cancer has spread to the bladder, rectum, or other organs close to the cervix.
IV-B	Cancer has spread to distant organs such as the lungs.
Recurrent	The cancer has come back, in the cervix or elsewhere, after treatment.

Most patients with stage I and stage II-A cancers can be cured, but the higher the stage, the more intensive the therapy. That's why staging is such an important, though often exhausting, procedure.

One more point about that *New Yorker* article: The story about the unfortunate young woman with ASCUS on her Pap smear and a diagnosis of cervical cancer has a rather awful ending—she dies of her disease. And as I said earlier, about five thousand women die of cervical cancer every year in the United States. That's five thousand too many, and that's the bad news about cervical cancer. Remember, though, that about fourteen thousand new cases of cervical cancer are diagnosed every year, so the good news is that most women diagnosed with cervical cancer survive it. In other words, although cervical cancer is potentially fatal, most cases are diagnosed at an early, curable stage. The message? If you have an abnormal Pap smear, or if you exhibit any of the symptoms mentioned above, you need to be followed up as soon as possible. The second is that if you *are* given a diagnosis of cervical cancer, in most cases, chances are that you will beat it and live a long, healthy life!

Staging usually starts with blood and urine tests. Next, your physician will perform a thorough pelvic exam with you under anesthesia, and he or she may do a *cystoscopy* and *proctosigmoidoscopy*. In a cystoscopy, she'll look inside your bladder with a thin, lighted instrument to check for cancerous areas; proctosigmoidoscopy uses the same procedure to look inside your rectum and lower large intestine. She may also order x-rays to check your bladder, rectum, lymph nodes, and lungs. A *computerized tomography* (CT), also known as a CAT scan, is useful for checking for enlarged lymph nodes and for other signs of cancer spread within or beyond the pelvis.

Once all the evidence is gathered and the stage of your

cancer is determined, a cancer specialist, often a gynecologic oncologist, will take your general and specific health
issues into consideration and decide on a treatment plan.
At this point, you may want to contact another gynecologic
oncologist for a second opinion to review both the diagnosis and treatment plan. Some insurance companies cover
second opinions, and others even *require* it. Although it
may delay the start of your treatment by a week or two, the
delay will not reduce the chance of successful treatment.
Your doctor can probably suggest physicians to consult,
and the Cancer Information service (1-800-4-CANCER) can
tell you about treatment facilities supported by the National
Cancer Institute. Another useful site for women with cervical cancer is sponsored by the American Cancer Society at
http://www.cancer.org/. In the future, clinical trials will
probably be available for all stages of cervical cancer. However, because the success rate is lower with standard therapy for stage III or IV cancer, you might especially want to
consider experimental therapies should you have cancer at
these advanced stages.

Treatment

Treatment for cervical cancer varies widely depending on
the stage, so I've organized this section according to stage.

Stage 0

This stage is known as "precancer" or carcinoma in situ,
which I covered in chapter 6. As you know, this isn't really

invasive cancer. You won't even need staging at this point; a colposcopy will indicate that the abnormal cells are still located above the basement membrane. Procedures like LEEP and conization remove all of the abnormal cells, and recurrence is relatively rare.

Stage I-A

At this early stage, the cancer has only just begun to invade deeper tissues. The most commonly recommended treatment at this point is a hysterectomy, in which the cervix and uterus are removed. Depending on the depth of the invasion, internal radiation therapy may also be considered. If the cancer is localized enough, conization is another, less traumatic option for cancer removal. A *trachelectomy* is a new alternative to hysterectomy. All of these options are described later in this chapter.

Stage I-B

Stage I-B cancer describes cancer that is more extensive than that seen with stage I-A, but still hasn't spread beyond the cervix into the surrounding tissues. With more intensive therapy than that of stage I-A, most cases can be cured. Treatment may include one of the following options: internal and external radiation therapy; radical hysterectomy with lymph node dissection; radical hysterectomy and lymph node dissection followed by radiation therapy plus chemotherapy; or radiation therapy plus chemotherapy alone. All of these options are described later in this chapter.

Stage II-A

The cancer has spread beyond the cervix and has invaded the upper two-thirds of your vagina at this point. It's usually treated in the same manner as Stage I-B cervical cancer.

Stage II-B

At this stage, the cancerous cells have spread to the tissues surrounding the cervix and require combined internal and external radiation therapy combined with chemotherapy.

Stage III

This stage requires the same treatment as II-B, but because cancer has spread throughout much of the pelvic area, and cancer cells may have spread to the lower part of the vagina, the treatment will probably take longer, with a lower success rate.

Stage IV-A

Again, therapy at this stage usually consists of combined internal and external radiation with chemotherapy, with a longer, more intensive treatment. Because the cancer has spread to the bladder, rectum, or other organs close to the cervix, those organs will require radiation as well.

Stage IV-B

Because the cancer has spread to other parts of the body such as the lungs, this stage of cancer is usually not considered curable. Treatment—usually including radiation and chemotherapy—is considered *palliative*, which means symptom-relieving, but not curative, and designed to make the patient feel more comfortable.

Recurrent Cancer

Recurrent cancer (cancer that has come back) also involves palliative radiation and chemotherapy. At this point, depending on where the cancer returned and how extensive the tumor is, patients may be eligible for potentially curative radical surgery or clinical trials (described later in this chapter).

Treatment Options for Cervical Cancer

Hysterectomy

As a rule, the word *hysterectomy* can be as frightening as *cancer*, despite its curative nature. For a woman, the removal of some of her reproductive organs is traumatic and even tragic, especially if she planned on having children. Although it may seem like a drastic measure, the alternatives are usually deemed so much less attractive that hysterectomy is preferable. The primary argument against having a hysterectomy is that it removes the possibility of pregnancy, but the alternatives—radiation and chemotherapy—can also cause long-term fertility problems.

Several kinds of hysterectomies exist, and the selection of which type depends on how far the cancer has spread. The most common surgery for women in Stage I-A is a *total hysterectomy*, which removes the cervix, uterus, and fallopian tubes. In women under the age of forty, the ovaries are left intact to continue producing estrogen, although some women still show signs of menopause following a total hysterectomy.

If you're past the age of forty, your doctor will probably choose to remove the ovaries as well. This is called *total abdominal hysterectomy with bilateral salpingo-oophorectomy* (TAH-BSO). In that case, you'll begin hormone replacement therapy while you're still in the hospital to lessen the effects of surgical menopause, an unfortunate but inevitable side effect of this procedure.

If your tumor has a deeper invasion (3 to 5 millimeters), your specialist may choose to perform a radical hysterectomy with lymph node dissection. This surgery removes the cancer, the uterus, cervix, part of the vagina, and the lymph nodes in the pelvic area. Removal of the lymph nodes helps to determine if the cancer has already been spread to this area and helps to prevent further spread. Again, you'll begin hormone replacement immediately to curb the surgical menopause.

How a Hysterectomy Is Done

Today, there are several methods for performing a hysterectomy, and your physician will consider the state of your general health and the extent of the cancer in deciding which route to take.

The most common form of hysterectomy is *abdominal*, in which the organs are removed through an incision in your abdomen. Like a cesarean section incision, it's about six to eight inches long in the lower abdomen, and runs either vertically (from the belly button to the pubic bone) or horizontally (the "bikini cut"). Following the surgery, your hospitalization will last three or four days, and total recovery takes four to six weeks. You'll be advised as to how long you should wait to resume sexual relations, but the usual recommendation is four weeks.

A newer method of hysterectomy is *vaginal*, in which the uterus is removed through the vagina. Though the recovery time is considerably shorter than for abdominal hysterectomy, this method can lead to discomfort during sexual intercourse due to shortening or tightening of the vagina. If the cancer has spread further than the uterus, vaginal hysterectomy is not an option.

After a Hysterectomy

Most complications of hysterectomy are the same as in any routine surgery. Antibiotics decrease the risk of infection from surgery. About 10 percent of women will require a blood transfusion due to preexisting anemia, and virtually all women feel tired in the days following their surgery.

Many women experience urinary tract infections, which are easily treated with antibiotics, and the cutting of sensory nerves during surgery can sometimes result in urinary incontinence. Postoperative bleeding typically lasts from several days to several weeks after surgery, with occasional spotting after intercourse or physical activity. Bleeding that occurs later than two months after your surgery could be caused by anything from granulation tissue (healing tissue growing on its own) to a return of the cancer. In either case, a pelvic exam is the best way to determine the source of the bleeding.

Other postoperative symptoms that may occur in the first two weeks include incisional problems (bloating, a healing itch, discharge from the incision, localized pain); gastrointestinal problems (increased gas, constipation, or loose stools); vaginal problems (discharge, odor, vulvar burning or itching due to dryness); pelvic cramps; or general allergy symptoms due to antibiotics or pain medications. Many of these symptoms can be treated with over-the-counter products or prescription medication.

As far as resuming normal activities, take it easy for four to six weeks. You've had major surgery, and your body needs to recuperate. Return to your daily activities in short bursts after the first forty-eight hours: Resting for forty minutes out of every hour in the first two weeks is a good system. If any activity causes excessive pain, stop doing it. Ease into heavy physical activity; abdominal exercises may be resumed at six weeks—but again, *ease* into it. Don't just rest in bed for six weeks, though. The earlier you resume physical activity (in short bursts), the better shape you'll be in when you're fully healed.

In addition to these postoperative symptoms, many women experience emotional and sexual side effects of hysterectomy. A primary fear is that you'll lose your sex drive after the hysterectomy, but that's often more related to emotional rather than physiological problems. You *do* need to wait until your doctor gives you the OK to have sex—before you're healed, sex may be painful and could potentially slow your recovery—but once he or she says you're in the clear, go for it.

Your vagina, not your cervix, produces the lubrication for sex, and your vagina is *not* removed in a hysterectomy. You will still be fully capable of having an orgasm, and although some feelings may be different (for instance, during orgasm some women experience a tightening in the cervix, which will no longer occur), your ability to achieve orgasm won't decrease. You may experience some vaginal dryness, a problem easily remedied by K-Y jelly or any vaginal lubricant. Some women may experience pain during sexual intercourse at first owing to the sensitivity of the area and the possible tightening of the vaginal wall.

If your ovaries are removed as well, menopause will begin to occur immediately following the surgery, and hormone replacement therapy is usually integrated into your recovery routine. The ovaries are rarely removed in women under forty, but for women close to menopause, physicians commonly opt to remove the ovaries (*oophorectomy* in medicalese). A decrease in ovary-produced estrogen may cause a decrease in sexual desire, true, but hormonal treatment can offset the effects of surgical menopause.

Often, women may feel undesirable or somehow "less womanly" without a complete set of reproductive organs. In addition, the knowledge that childbearing is no longer an option can be traumatic to younger women. But many women are relieved that their worries about cancer are over: Now they can lead a full, healthy, cancer-free life. In addition, support groups for hysterectomy patients exist

both in your community and online. (See the section entitled "Online Support Groups" in appendix D.)

You do need to continue getting Pap smears after a
hysterectomy, despite the loss of your cervix. A Pap can
also show abnormalities in the vagina, and you'll need to
continue getting checkups to confirm the absence of cancer cells.

Internal Radiation Therapy

For patients who cannot undergo surgery, *internal radiation therapy* (also called *intracavitary radiation therapy*) may be prescribed. Radiation therapy uses penetrating
beams of high-energy waves of radiation to kill abnormal
cells. Because cancer cells grow and divide faster than normal cells, but are weaker than healthy cells, radiation pref-
erentially kills or prevents cancer cells from dividing.
Normal cells are affected by radiation as well, but most of
them recover from the effects. Doctors take measures to
protect normal cells from the radiation by limiting the dose
of radiation, spreading the treatment out over time, and
shielding as much normal tissue as possible during therapy.

Like surgery, radiation therapy is considered to be
"local," since it only targets cells in the affected part of the
body. If you're still in the first stages of cervical cancer,
your doctor may use it after your surgery to kill any remaining cancer cells.

Internal radiation therapy uses higher concentrations of
radiation than external radiation therapy. Instead of using a
large radiation machine, the radioactive material (usually
cesium, iridium, iodine, phosphorous, or palladium) is

sealed in a thin wire, catheter, or implant and placed directly into the affected tissue. This method decreases radiation damage to the surrounding normal tissue and takes less time than external therapy.

How Internal Radiation Therapy for Cervical Cancer Is Done

To treat cervical cancer with internal radiation therapy, a container of the radioactive material is placed in your cervix; your doctor may or may not choose to remove the capsule after your therapy is finished. When left in place, the radioactive substance loses potency quickly and becomes nonradioactive.

In the hospital, you'll be given a local or general anesthesia so that you won't feel pain when your doctor fixes the applicator in place. If the implant feels uncomfortable for you, you'll probably be prescribed muscle relaxers or pain relievers; you may have to lie still to prevent it from shifting inside you. Make sure you tell your nurse about any side effects you experience.

Although the radiation therapy is helping you, it's dangerous for others, so the hospital will take measures to protect staff and visitors from its effects.

You'll probably stay in a private room, and nurses will spend only short amounts of time with you during your therapy. Visitors under age eighteen and pregnant women will not be able to visit you, and most visitors will probably have to sit six feet from your bed. You may also have a rolling lead shield beside your bed to place between you and visitors or staff. While the experience can be lonely and unpleasant, it usually only lasts for one to three days at a time over a period of two weeks at the most.

Removal of the implant is a quick procedure, and you probably won't even require an anesthetic. You're no longer radioactive at that point, so your visitors are unlimited. Once you leave the hospital, you should be able to resume activity immediately, with short breaks for resting periods. You may be sore or sensitive for a few days, and your doctor will probably tell you to limit sexual activities for a while after therapy.

After Internal Radiation Therapy

Hair loss is a common side effect of radiation treatment. However, because the radiation is usually concentrated in the pelvic region, this is an uncommon side effect of treatment for cervical cancer. Conversely, because the radiation therapy is located in your pelvis, you may experience nausea and a loss of appetite. However, it's important that you keep up your caloric intake for strength. You may also experience bladder irritation and painful or frequent urination; drinking plenty of fluids usually helps. You may also stop menstruating and experience vaginal itching, burning, and dryness. If the radiation reaches your bowels, you may experience diarrhea, pain, and bleeding with bowel movements. Your doctor or nurse can suggest treatment for these symptoms.

Sexual intercourse may be painful or uncomfortable during the first few weeks after radiation therapy, but those symptoms should disappear after three weeks at the most. Some women may notice a decrease in sexual desire, but that may be due to stress and fatigue in addition to any side effects from the radiation. Some women also experience shrinkage in the vaginal tissues, in which case you may want to use a dilator (a device that gently stretches your vaginal tissue).

Scientists are still studying the effects of radiation on fertility, and it's an issue you should discuss at length with your doctor. Radiation therapy during pregnancy (especially during the first trimester) may injure the fetus and is strongly discouraged. Long-term effects on fertility may occur as well.

Follow-up care is necessary to deal with any side effects of radiation, as well as to detect any trace or recurring signs of cancer. This type of care can include more cancer treatments, rehabilitation, counseling, and returning to see the radiation oncologist. You may go to your primary-care doctor as well. Always, always, follow any instructions from either doctor, and work hard at keeping up your general health: Eat a balanced diet and resume exercise and regular daily activities as soon as possible.

External Radiation Therapy

External radiation therapy utilizes the same concept as internal—using radioactive material to kill weak, abnormal cells—but it does not involve any kind of implant within your body. It's the more common form of therapy and usually occurs during outpatient visits to a hospital or treatment center. A machine directs high-energy rays at the cancer and a small margin of the tissues surrounding it.

How External Radiation Therapy Is Done

The most common type of machine for external radiation therapy is called a linear accelerator. The machines use a variety of radioactive substances (X-rays, electron beams, or cobalt-60 gamma rays), and the oncologist will decide the best one for your cervical cancer.

The first step in external radiation therapy is called *simulation*. You'll lie very still on a table while an X-ray machine defines your ideal treatment ports, the exact place where the radiation will be aimed. CT scans and other imaging may also be used to plan the direction of the radiation. Immobilization devices such as body molds may be created at this time to keep you from moving during treatment. In fact, it's so important that the radiation is targeted exactly the same every time that your radiation therapist will even mark your treatment ports with tiny dots of permanent ink.

Based on your medical history, lab tests, X-rays, and other treatments you've had, your doctor and radiation therapist will decide how much radiation is needed, what kind of machine to use, and how many treatments you should have. Any of these factors could vary during your therapy, depending on how well you're responding to the treatment.

During your visits, you'll change into a hospital gown or robe. Your therapist will position you for optimal exposure of your treatment ports; you'll probably be lying down on a table or sitting in a special chair. The therapist may place shields around other parts of your body to block the radiation from surrounding tissue. You must try to hold completely still during the treatment.

The radiation therapist leaves the room before treatment begins and will watch and listen to you during your entire therapy. At first, the therapy may seem frightening—

the machines are large, move around you, and make noises—but keep in mind that the therapist is always watching you as he or she controls the machines, and can stop the treatment at any time if you ask.

Each session lasts about fifteen to thirty minutes, with about one to five of those minutes devoted to radiation, which is undetectable—you won't hear, smell, taste, see, or feel the radiation. Depending on your doctor's orders, you'll probably have therapy five days a week for six to seven weeks.

After your treatment, you can go home, although you will likely suffer unpleasant side effects. They'll go away within a few weeks of your last treatment, although some can last longer. Many can be managed with medication.

Side Effects of External Radiation Therapy

Side effects vary greatly from person to person, depending on the level of radiation used and your general health. *Acute* side effects occur soon after the start of treatment and usually fade after a few weeks. *Chronic* side effects may develop after months or years and many are permanent.

Two of the most common acute side effects are fatigue and alterations in your skin at the site of radiation treatment, ranging from very dry, itchy, sunburned-looking skin to a moist, wet reaction. Dry skin can be treated with ointments, and you should notify your doctor of a moist reaction, since the area can become infected. Don't rub or scrub the area or wear tight clothing over it, and use very mild soap with lukewarm water for cleansing.

Fatigue is the most common symptom. Your body will

use a lot of energy for healing during radiation therapy. If you're experiencing a low appetite, lowered blood counts, and the general stress involved with treatment, it all adds up to one very tired woman. You may want to try some light exercise like walking, and if you have a full-time job, take some time off or work reduced hours. Save your energy for the most important tasks, like getting well! Other side effects may include nausea, hair loss, bladder irritation, and other pelvic symptoms outlined previously.

After External Radiation Therapy

As with internal therapy, always talk to your doctor about any long-lasting, excessive side effects. Effects of the therapy should go away within a few weeks of the last treatment. Be sure to attend all of your follow-up examinations and ease into regular activities.

Chemotherapy

One of the most exciting developments in recent years has been the "new standard of care": a combination of chemotherapy and radiation therapy that cuts the mortality rate of cervical cancer in half. Chemotherapy, or chemical therapy, uses drugs to kill cancer cells, and is most often used when the cancer has spread to other parts of the body. Unlike radiation or surgery, it isn't localized. It's systemic, meaning it affects the entire body. The drugs are designed to destroy cancer cells by stopping them from growing or multiplying, but they can also damage healthy cells—especially the ones that divide quickly, which is what causes side effects. Recently cisplatin-based drugs have been used increasingly for treatment for cervical cancer. Several recent trials have shown that women who undergo combination therapy with cisplatin have better survival rates than when they have radiation therapy alone. Sometimes cisplatin is given in combination with another chemotherapy drug we've discussed before: 5-fluorouracil (5-FU, or Efedux). In this case, the 5-fluorouracil is given intravenously instead of in a cream form applied to the skin.

Who should consider chemotherapy? Patients who have big tumors at the stage I-B and II-A phase may add it to their radiation treatments. Patients who have stage II-B, III, and IV-A cancer and above should definitely consider adding it. Patients who have stage IV-B might consider other treatment combinations such as cisplatin with paclitaxel or cisplatin with gemcitabine. For stage IV-B, many different treatment trials are in progress.

How Chemotherapy Is Done

Chemotherapy can be administered in different settings, including your home, your doctor's office, a clinic, or as an outpatient or inpatient in a hospital. Most often, you'll get "chemo" as an outpatient, possibly with a short initial stay to monitor side effects.

The drugs can be administered in several different ways: intravenously (IV), through injection, or by mouth. With IV treatment, your doctor or nurse will insert a needle into a vein, usually in your arm, and the drugs will be dripped through the duration of your session. Another option is a catheter, a tube that is left in your vein for as long as necessary so you don't have to have a new needle inserted every time. By mouth, the drug is in a pill or capsule form and is taken like any other oral drug.

Depending on the stage of your cancer, the intensity and duration of chemo may vary. Chemo is always administered in cycles: treatment followed by recovery, then more treatment followed by another recovery period.

Side Effects of Chemotherapy

Because chemo can also damage other quickly dividing cells, many patients experience side effects related to their digestive tract, reproductive system, and hair follicles. Of course, the exact side effects will vary with the specific chemotherapy drugs. The most common side effects of cisplatin are nausea, vomiting, and damage to the kidneys. Cisplatin may also reduce your fertility. Rarer side effects include damage to the bone marrow, which might result in anemia, easy bruisability, and decreased ability to fight off infections. Women may also experience numbness and tingling in their hands and feet, diarrhea, ringing in the ears, a change in the taste in their mouth, and loss of appetite. The most common side effects of 5-fluorouracil include nausea and vomiting, sores in the mouth, diarrhea, and damage to the bone marrow. Hair thinning, changes to nails, changes in vision, sensitivity to sunlight, and rashes can also occur with 5-fluorouracil. Some of these side effects are discussed in greater detail below.

As with radiation, the most common symptom is fatigue, caused by your body's natural healing process, stress, and a host of other factors. Chemo-related fatigue is more severe than everyday tiredness. It can come on suddenly and you may feel a total lack of energy that simple bed rest can't relieve.

Nausea and vomiting have also been common side effects of chemo, although combining antiemetic (antinausea) drugs with chemo can greatly lessen them. Work with your doctor in finding the best combination for you, and be patient: You may have to try several drugs before finding relief. Try drinking liquids an hour before or after meals, instead of with food. Eat and drink slowly and eat small meals of dry food. Try to distract yourself by chatting with friends or watching television. If your nausea is still so severe that you can't keep down liquids, talk with your doctor about adjusting your treatment.

Diarrhea is another unpleasant digestive side effect of chemo. The most important thing to remember with diarrhea is to replenish your fluids: Watery or loose stools can empty your body of much-needed fluids and nutrients, and if it persists, your doctor may give you an IV to replace what you've lost. Drink only clear or light fluids like ginger ale; avoid caffeine and dairy products. If your therapy causes constipation, drink plenty of water, try exercising, and eat high-fiber foods.

Chemo can also damage nerves, causing dull to intense pain in some patients. Describe your pain to your caregivers in as much detail as possible so that you can receive the appropriate treatment—many drugs exist to control cancer pain, and we want you to be as comfortable as possible during your treatment. Relaxation exercises also help distract you or lessen the tension of chemo.

Another common side effect is hair loss (*alopecia* in medicalese). Not all drugs cause alopecia, and alopecia is not a common side effect of cisplatin and 5-FU. Your doctor will tell you beforehand if you're taking a chemotherapy drug that does cause alopecia. It can occur on all parts of the body, from your head to your pubic hair, but it usually grows back after the treatment ends. You may want to cut your hair short before chemo to make the difference seem less dramatic, or wear a wig or scarf if you feel self-conscious. Although usually painless, hair loss can be a traumatic experience for many women. Feelings of anger or depression are common, but remember that hair loss is only temporary: Your hair *will* grow back.

Chemotherapy can also damage the cells of the bone marrow, and you'll need to be monitored for this with blood tests. It results in anemia, caused by a reduction in your bone marrow's ability to make red blood cells. Your red blood cells carry nutrients and oxygen throughout your body, and without them, your body has to work much harder to accomplish smaller tasks. You may feel tired or short of breath. Your doctor will check your blood frequently during chemo, and if anemia persists, he or she may prescribe drugs or even a blood transfusion to boost your red blood cell count.

You can also help by eating a well-balanced diet, limiting your activities, and getting plenty of rest. Since the bone marrow also contains platelets (cells important for blood clotting) and white blood cells (cells important for fighting off infection), chemotherapy may also lead to increased risk of bleeding and infections. If you notice increased bruising, bleeding that won't stop easily, or new red spots on your skin, you should notify your doctor immediately. Also, if you notice a fever, or if you feel ill for any reason, you need to notify your doctor immediately.

Chemo can also reduce the hormones produced by your ovaries, resulting in irregular and absent periods during treatment. This effect can be temporary or permanent. Similarly, the drugs could cause temporary or permanent infertility and/or menopause. Some women only experience menopausal symptoms such as hot flashes or vaginal dryness, while others run the course of full menopause. Vaginal and bladder infections may increase, as well, and you may find intercourse uncomfortable. Some anticancer drugs can cause birth defects, so chemo during pregnancy is not advisable. See the section entitled "Pregnancy and Cervical Cancer" on page 179.

Coping with Chemo

Though it often provides a cure for cervical cancer, chemo can be a stressful, unpleasant, painful process. It disrupts your routine, your general health, and your hormones, and is a source of stress to yourself and the people around you. Feeling angry or depressed is only natural.

In addition to the people around you like your family, friends, doctors and nurses, you may want to seek out counseling professionals for help in expressing and coping with your feelings during treatment and, indeed, during the entire cancer ordeal. Support groups for current and past chemo patients can be enormously helpful. They're usually attended by people who are going through what you are or who have been through it, and who are probably experiencing the same painful emotions and side effects as you. Whether they come in the form of online bulletin boards or whether it's a formal group of people, support groups are important sources of practical information and can even improve your recovery physically. Your doctor or clinic can recommend local groups.

Clinical Trials

Scientists are constantly developing and testing new drugs and therapies, so you may choose to be part of a *clinical trial*. After the long, careful process of cancer research, doctors test the most promising approaches to prevention, diagnosis, and treatment on volunteers.

Clinical trials are a wonderful opportunity for you and your doctor to try a new approach to prevention, treatment, or even your own comfort. All trials include their own sets of risks and benefits, though, so always discuss your choice with your doctor. Make sure you understand all the pros and cons before committing to one.

Types of Trials

Screening, or diagnosis, trials test new ways to catch early stages of cervical cancer as well as improve the staging process (like the Pap smear and the HPV DNA test). Similar trials may also test new ways to catch HSIL, moderate or severe dysplasia.

Prevention trials test medicines, vitamins, minerals, and other supplements to lower the risk of developing cervical cancer, and if you've already had cancer, to prevent recurrence. Of course, the most effective prevention for dysplasia and cancer would be to avoid initial infection with HPV, or to be vaccinated against HPV; HPV vaccines are in clinical trials right now.

Treatment trials include new chemotherapy drugs, methods of radiation, gene therapy, and combinations. The recent combination of chemo and radiation therapy is a direct result of successful clinical trials and has become the new standard of cervical cancer care. Trials are also in progress to use vaccines against HPV as a form of therapy, and not just prevention of infection as I mentioned above.

A fourth kind of trial, for **quality of life**, is of particular help to stage IV cervical cancer patients and patients with recurrent cervical cancer, but can help earlier stages too. Also called **supportive care** trials, they test ways to improve your life during treatment and recovery (anti-nausea drugs, the effects of alternative care, etc.).

Most trials progress in a series of phases:

Phase I trials study how a new drug should be administered (by mouth, injection into blood or muscle, etc.), how often, and which dose is safe. These trials are usually the smallest, enrolling as few as a dozen patients at a time.

Phase II trials tests the safety of a drug and evaluate how well it works.

Phase III trials test a new drug and compare the results against the current standard. Participants are assigned to a control group (the current standard of care) or test group (new care) at random; the groups are much larger than in phase I or phase II trials and may be conducted at many centers nationwide. Phase III trials primarily focus on how well the new drug or approach works, but safety is an important focus as well.

How Can I Get Involved?

Because clinical trials are a part of a scientific study, the criteria for participation are usually quite strict. Participants are generally alike in a particular way, such as similar stage of cancer, age, gender, or previous treatments. Clinical trials are usually conducted at a larger cancer center, a university hospital, or occasionally in your local hospital or physician's office. The National Cancer Institute (on the campus of the National Institutes of Health in Bethesda, Maryland) also conducts frequent clinical trials.

Two Web sites supported by the National Institutes of Health list different available clinical trials should you wish to consider participating in a research study.

- *http://clinicaltrials.gov/ct/gui/c/b*
- *www.cancer.gov/search/clinical_trials*

Depending on the type of trial—treatment, supportive, etc.—you may have to travel to one or two highly specialized centers. During the trial, you'd be under supervision and guidance of a team of health professionals and your experience would be reported back to the center conducting the trial. During and after the trial, experts evaluate the results. Keep in mind, though, that your health insurance may not cover the cost of a clinical trial since they're often considered "experimental" or "investigational" procedures.

When you enroll in a clinical trial, you're giving your *informed consent*. That means you understand all the key facts about the trial before participating: the reason for the study, the nature of the intervention in the trial, risks and benefits, and the tests you may have. *Ask questions about everything.* If you're unsure about anything, ask your doctor or the trial team—this is your health, so you deserve to know all the facts.

The National Cancer Institute suggests asking your doctor these questions before participating:

The Study

- What is the purpose of the study?
- Why do researchers think the approach may be effective?
- Who will sponsor the study?
- Who has reviewed and approved the study?
- How are study results and safety of participants being checked?
- How long will the study last?
- How long will each visit last?
- What are my responsibilities if I participate?

Possible Risks and Benefits

- What are my possible short-term benefits?
- What are my possible long-term benefits?
- What are my short-term risks, such as side effects? Loss of privacy?
- What are my possible long-term risks?
- What other options do people with my risk of cancer or type of cancer have?
- How do the possible risks and benefits of this trial compare with those options?

Participation and Care

- What kinds of therapies, procedures, and/or tests will I have during the trial?
- Will they hurt, and if so, for how long?

- How do the tests in the study compare with those I would have outside of the trial?
- Will I be able to take my regular medications while in the clinical trial?
- Where will I have my medical care?
- Who will be in charge of my care?

Personal Issues

- How could being in this study affect my daily life?
- Can I talk to other people in the study?

Cost Issues

- Will I have to pay for any part of the trial such as tests or the study drug?
- If so, what will the charges likely be?
- What is my health insurance likely to cover?
- Who can help answer any questions from my insurance company or health plan?
- Will there be any travel or child care costs that I need to consider while I am in the trial?

Tips for Asking Your Doctor about Trials

When you talk with your doctor or members of the research team:

- Consider taking a family member or friend along for support and for help in asking questions or recording answers.
- Plan ahead what to ask—but don't hesitate to ask any new questions you think of while you're there.
- Write down your questions in advance to make sure you remember to ask them all.
- Write down the answers so that you can review them whenever you want.

Source: http://cancertrials.nci.nih.gov/understanding/participating/questions.html

Fertility and Cervical Cancer

While eradicating the cancer and most likely preventing its recurrence, hysterectomies render a woman incapable of ever having a child. For many young women, this can be a tragic side effect of cervical cancer.

A new surgery could be changing all that. Available only in Canada at the time of this writing, the new *radical trachelectomy* removes only the cervix, not the uterus. The surgery is usually done in conjunction with a pelvic lymph node dissection to prevent spread of cancer cells. The surgery is *not* for patients over age forty, and it's only for earlier stages of cervical cancer. Thus far the rate of recurrence is comparable to that of hysterectomy. Some infertility still occurs despite the surgery, and late miscarriages occur in about a fourth of trachelectomy patients. However, the rate of pregnancy after surgery is about 40 percent. That may seem low, but compared with the 0 percent pregnancy rate of hysterectomy, trachelectomy offers an exciting alternative and hope for young cancer patients (Covens et al. 1999). Keep in mind, though, that studies on trachelectomies are very new, and only limited data exist on the long-term cervical cancer recurrence rate.

Radiation and chemotherapy can both significantly reduce fertility, although many young women have chosen to preserve a portion of their ovaries for cryopreservation (freezing eggs to preserve them). A technique for collecting ovarian tissue (known as *laparoscopy*) has been proven to be a safe, effective method for preserving eggs. In this technique, a thin instrument called a laparoscope is inserted directly into the belly and the ovarian eggs are collected. If you undergo combination chemo and radiation therapy instead of a hysterectomy, there is a possibility that preserving your eggs could result in a later pregnancy. This approach is also in its early stages, though, and requires more study (Meirow et al. 1999).

Pregnancy and Cervical Cancer

The primary dilemma when a pregnant woman learns that she has cervical cancer is: *Should I defer treatment? Or should I start treatment immediately?* The answers to those questions depend on the stages of both the pregnancy and the cancer, and can involve some painful choices by a woman and her spouse or partner.

The traditional approach has been to recommend therapy appropriate to the stage of disease and to delay therapy only if the cancer is detected in the third trimester. However, some reports suggest that if you're in the first stages of cancer—Stage I-A or I-B—it might be possible to delay therapy until an improved fetal outcome can be assured. Chemotherapy can be extremely damaging to a fetus, and early radiation can cause both malformations and mental retardation.

If you're still in the first trimester and your doctor is concerned the cancer could harm either you or the baby before carrying to full term, you may have to consider ending the pregnancy and undergoing a hysterectomy. The choice can be difficult, but you, your partner, and your doctor can decide together what's best for you and your family.

Conclusion

I've given you a lot of information in this one chapter, and you may feel a bit overwhelmed. You probably realize, though, that a single book could be written about any of these topics—radiation therapy, chemotherapy, hysterectomies, cervical cancer—and, in fact, many books on these subjects already exist. Before engaging in any treatment, discuss your options with your doctor; ultimately, your health is in your own hands.

Coping with cancer—and especially cancer of a personal area like the cervix—will be a difficult experience, both emotionally and physically. No two women are exactly like, so no two women will experience the same reactions to treatment. Your doctor knows your health history the best, so he or she will be the best one to discuss your prognosis with you.

The outlook for women in the precancerous or early stages of cancer is excellent. Nearly all patients through stage II-A can be cured. The new combination of chemo and radiation therapy is encouraging. Not only does it cut the mortality rate for more advanced cervical cancer in half, but it also gives hope for the constantly emerging new treatments and therapies in treating cervical cancer.

In the meantime, hundreds of support groups for

women like you exist: Hysterectomy, chemo, radiation, and cervical cancer patients all have forums, especially on the Web. Any hospital or clinic can probably recommend some local groups for you, and your doctor is sure to know a few offhand.

PART THREE

Anogenital Dysplasias in Areas Other Than the Cervix: Vagina, Vulva, and Anus

CHAPTER EIGHT

Vaginal Dysplasia and Cancer

Although cervical cancer is the most publicized, common cancer caused by HPV infection, it's by no means the only one. Several other cancers have been directly connected to HPV. Vaginal cancer is one of these.

The vagina is subject to all kinds of trauma: At any point, it may contain a penis, finger, tampon, vibrator, or baby. It opens up to the outside of the body, so it's prone to developing irritations like bacterial vaginosis and yeast infections. In general, though, it's a strong organ, and self-cleansing; it usually produces the amount of mucus it needs to rid itself of bacteria and imbalances, whether "heavy" or "light." As we know, though, lowered immunity, previous infections, age, and general health can affect any part of a woman's anatomy, and HPV infection can take advantage of those weaknesses and eventually lead to vaginal cancer. Figure 2.1 shows the vagina and where it sits between the cervix and vulva.

Vaginal cancer, while more common than vulvar cancer, is still relatively rare. These are cancers that comprise 1 to 2 percent of all gynecologic malignancies. There are two types: squamous cell cancer and adenocarcinoma. That just means they affect different types of cells: squamous cells, the flat skin-surface cells I mentioned earlier; and "adeno," or glandular cells, like the ones that line the endocervical canal, which produce fluids and hormones in the body. Just as there is squamous cell cancer and adenocarcinoma of the cervix, the vagina can be the site of both of these kinds of cancer. The distinction between vaginal squamous cell carcinoma and vaginal adenocarcinoma is important—they have different causes, natural history, and treatment. Vaginal adenocarcinomas are usually found in "DES daughters," women whose mothers took diethylstilbestrol (DES) during their pregnancy to prevent miscarriages.

About 85 percent of all vaginal cancers are the squamous cell type. They're often, but not always, found in association with the same HPV types linked with cancer of the cervix. Like the outer part of the cervix, the vagina is lined by squamous epithelium; like the cervical squamous epithelium, the vaginal epithelium is at risk of HPV infection. But for the same reasons that the outer layer of the cervix is less vulnerable than the "transformation zone" of the cervix—because there's not as much cell activity—the vaginal epithelium is at relatively low risk of infection when compared to the cervical transformation zone. Oncogenic HPV infection can and does, however, cause vaginal cancer.

Vaginal squamous cell cancer is found most often in women between the ages of sixty and eighty. It initially spreads superficially within the vaginal wall and later invades the underlying tissues and adjacent organs. If it metastasizes, it usually goes to the lungs and liver. It may develop as a result of HPV reactivation due to age-related loss of immunity and lack of health care.

As I described in chapter 1, the minor trauma and abrasions that occur during sex may provide entry into the basal cells of the vagina, allowing HPV to take hold and replicate.

Just as cervical cancer is preceded by dysplasia, vaginal cancer may be preceded by a lesion known as *vaginal intraepithelial neoplasia* (VAIN). Just as in the cervix, we throw around a lot of terms that essentially mean the same thing, so another word for VAIN is vaginal dysplasia. Although we don't usually use the term in the context of the vagina, these are also squamous intraepithelial lesions. And although the vagina lacks the transformation zone of the cervix, thus lessening the chances of serious infection, HPV-associated VAIN is an increasingly common problem, most likely as a result of more widespread HPV infection.

A word of caution: As you now know, the relationship between HPV, cervical dysplasia, and cervical cancer is close. Almost all cervical dysplasia is associated with HPV, and we believe almost all cervical cancers arise from dysplasia. Not surprisingly, almost all cervical cancers are associated with HPV.

The HPV-vaginal cancer link isn't quite as straightforward. Not all vaginal cancers are associated with HPV, and not all vaginal cancers arise from vaginal dysplasia. Having said that, we still have to treat vaginal dysplasia, since it definitely *can* progress to cancer.

In contrast to the squamous cell cancers, vaginal adeno-carcinomas are associated with DES use by the patient's mother during pregnancy. They're most often diagnosed in women between seventeen and twenty-one years of age and tend to be more aggressive; they spread more often to the lungs and lymph nodes around the body. Not surprisingly, this type of cancer is not usually associated with HPV.

Vaginal Dysplasia (Vaginal Intraepithelial Neoplasia, or VAIN)

First, I'd like to mention a few words about terminology again. Obviously, you might confuse the term *VAIN* (for "vaginal intraepithelial neoplasia") with *VIN*, which actually stands for "*vulvar* intraepithelial neoplasia." VAIN affects the vagina, and VIN affects the vulva. Just remember that the word *vagina* begins with the letters *va*, and you're set.

Vaginal dysplasia develops in much the same way as cervical dysplasia: HPV is introduced to the nucleus of a cell and the original cell divides, producing abnormal, HPV-infected progeny. The abnormal cells may create lesions known as dysplasia or neoplasia. In a small number of women, these can eventually lead to invasive cancer.

Symptoms of Vaginal Dysplasia

Vaginal dysplasia demonstrates few symptoms, although women who do self-examinations may notice bumps (*exophytic* lesions in medicalese) or warts. Vaginal dysplasia can be related to either high- or low-risk HPV types. If a high-risk type is introduced, exophytic warts *may* appear, but remember that many high-risk infections are also subclinical, so you may not notice any symptoms at all.

Diagnosis of Vaginal Dysplasia

A regular pelvic exam and Pap smear are the best defenses against vaginal dysplasia and vaginal cancer. Up to now, we've only talked about Pap smears to detect cervical disease, but they pick up vaginal disease too. (Haven't I been saying they're worth the time?) Cells picked up on a cervical Pap smear actually represent a mixture of both cervical cells and cells shed by the vaginal epithelium. So Pap smears may pick up vaginal abnormalities as well, and if your physician suspects that you have vaginal dysplasia, you'll probably be asked to come in for a colposcopy. (I outlined this process in chapter 4.)

The process for colposcopic examination is much the same for the vagina as for the cervix, and a pathologist will examine the biopsy. Your doctor usually freezes your tissue with a lidocaine injection to numb it, and uses biopsy forceps (similar to those used for cervical biopsies) to get a sample of vaginal tissue. After the biopsy, you may notice some bleeding and some discomfort once the anesthetic wears off.

Not surprisingly, if you have vaginal dysplasia, you're also at increased risk of having cervical lesions as well. In fact, you should think of HPV as a "field infection." If you're infected with HPV somewhere in the anogenital epithelium, there's a good chance it's also detectable elsewhere in the anogenital epithelium. You might even think of the anogenital epithelium as an "organ" in and of itself, and if HPV infection's a part of it, essentially the whole organ is affected. This doesn't mean HPV is detectable in every basal cell in the anogenital epithelium. Far from it—if HPV truly does affect the whole organ, it's likely to be patchy at best.

Staging and Treatment of Vaginal Dysplasia

If the biopsy shows that you have vaginal dysplasia, then by definition, you don't have cancer. As in the cervix, vaginal disease is staged as mild, moderate, and severe dysplasia: VAIN 1, 2, and 3, respectively, and pathologists use the same criteria to judge the lesions. As in the cervix, moderate and severe lesions need to be removed, while mild dysplasia could be treated, or at least monitored to make sure it goes away on its own.

Because vaginal dysplasia is less common than cervical dysplasia, we don't know as much about its natural history. But we assume the same rules apply: High-grade lesions have the potential to progress to cancer, while low-grade lesions have little or no potential to progress directly to cancer. Once again, as in the cervix, having mild dysplasia doesn't take you out of the woods, since some of these lesions can progress to moderate or severe dysplasia.

The treatment of vaginal dysplasia is based on the same principles as those for cervical disease: removal of the affected tissues by hook or by crook. In the vagina, there are many options to remove the lesions, and the choice depends on a number of factors: the size of the lesion, its location within the vagina, and the experience and preferences of your doctor.

LEEP

LEEP works on the walls of the vagina just as it does in the cervix. With LEEP, the lesion is scooped out with the electrical wire loop and sent for pathology, a primary advantage of the procedure.

Cost, however, is the main disadvantage of LEEP. On the other hand, LEEP is often a definitive treatment, and you won't have to return to your doctor's office as often as with other methods.

Following therapy, women often experience swelling and discomfort as well as a temporary change in the nature and quantity of vaginal discharge.

Laser Therapy

Some doctors prefer treating vaginal dysplasia with laser therapy, which uses a powerful light beam to destroy the abnormal tissue. Laser is used in the doctor's office, usually after a local anesthetic is applied. (General anesthesia is often used as well in day surgery settings.)

The main advantage of laser is its precision: The laser beam aims at the lesion to avoid hurting normal tissue, and your doctor can control the depth of the tissue destruction as well. The more superficial the destruction, the easier the healing process. The experience with laser varies from institution to institution, and in some, it's the treatment of choice for vaginal dysplasia.

As with all other treatment methods for vaginal dysplasia, lesion recurrence is a problem, mandating close follow-up.

Cold-Scalpel Excision

If the lesion is large, and invasive cancer can't be excluded, some doctors recommend surgical removal of the area. (This is the vaginal equivalent of the surgical cone biopsy for the cervix.) You'll go to a day surgery center, you'll be given an anesthetic, and the surgeon will remove wide areas of the vaginal epithelium for examination by a pathologist. Tissues not removed with the scalpel may also be treated with electrocautery, in which the doctor places a probe on the tissue, passes an electric current through it, and destroys the tissue.

Depending on the extent of the skin removal, skin grafting may be necessary to allow for complete healing.

Efudex (5-Fluorouracil) Cream

Efudex is a cream that contains the active ingredient 5-fluorouracil (5-FU). We've talked about 5-fluorouracil several times before. This compound is used for many different purposes other than treatment of vaginal dysplasia, including injection into the veins as a systemic chemotherapy agent for different kinds of cancer, including cervical cancer and colon cancer. For the purposes of treating vaginal dysplasia, though, 5-FU is applied to the surface of the lesion in a cream—one of those therapies you can do at home. Typically, a doctor will instruct you to apply the cream in a vaginal suppository once weekly for ten weeks, or in a more continuous fashion, such as three 7-day courses given one week apart.

As you might guess, the primary problem is that the 5-FU is *also* applied to normal tissue. Most of the time, this doesn't cause any problems, as long as too much cream doesn't make its way to these areas, but this therapeutic approach is essentially blind—once you insert it into your vagina, how do you know where the cream's going?

Unsurprisingly, a common complication is an ulcer or burn at one or more sites in the vagina. These can be painful and the healing may be accelerated with the use of zinc oxide creams. Because of these potential problems and because of the effectiveness of some of the other approaches mentioned above, 5-FU cream isn't used that often for treatment of vaginal dysplasia.

One important point to note: Since 5-FU cream works by damaging the cell's DNA, it should *not* be taken by pregnant women, because of the risk of harming the fetus.

Sexually active women who aren't pregnant must use effective contraception while using 5-FU cream.

Liquid Nitrogen

Liquid nitrogen therapy, also known as cryotherapy, is a less common approach to vaginal dysplasia treatment, and uses the same principle as cryotherapy for cervical disease. It is used primarily for treatment of mild dysplasia. Instead of placing a liquid-nitrogen–cooled probe onto the cervix to freeze the whole thing, the doctor directs the liquid nitrogen directly to the vaginal lesion in one of two ways. One way is to dip a swab into a vial of liquid nitrogen and then apply the (now extremely cold) swab tip directly to the surface of the lesion. Another way is to use a liquid nitrogen "gun," in which your doctor aims a stream of liquid nitrogen at the lesion. Often, the doctor applies the liquid nitrogen several times. Either way, the point is to freeze and kill the affected cells.

This procedure can be painful during application, but the pain usually fades soon after. Taking a painkiller such as ibuprofen or naproxen before the procedure might minimize the pain, and rarely, direct injection with 1 percent lidocaine is needed to provide adequate pain control.

Liquid nitrogen freezing works fairly well, but follow-up is necessary to make sure that the lesion is really gone and that it doesn't recur later. In many instances, you'll need multiple treatment attempts, with the treatment intervals ranging between one and three weeks.

Over a period of several days after the treatment, some swelling and discomfort may occur at the site of the lesion, and the dead tissue will slough off. During this time, you may note some discomfort with sexual intercourse and increase or change in your normal vaginal discharge.

Trichloroacetic Acid (TCA)

With liquid nitrogen, the tissue freezes to death. With TCA, the tissue burns with an acid: trichloroacetic acid. Like liquid nitrogen, TCA is used mostly for mild vaginal dysplasia. You'll notice that TCA has the word *acetic* in it, just like acetic acid or vinegar. Don't make the mistake of mixing these up, though—5 percent acetic acid is stuff we use to look for lesions in the cervix, and of course it's the stuff we put into our salads! In contrast, TCA is very nasty and can burn its way through practically anything. We apply it as carefully as possible to lesional areas only, and we *certainly* don't mix it with a little oil for our salads.

To treat the vaginal lesions with TCA, the doctor dips a stick or swab into a vial of the "vile" stuff and applies it directly to the lesion. Great effort is made to ensure that *only* the lesion is treated, since if the acid runs off, it could destroy the normal tissue as well. With TCA, we see the effect immediately—the lesion develops a dense white appearance. You'll *feel* the effect right away—when the treatment is working, you'll feel some heat at the site of the TCA application. Usually, it's uncomfortable but tolerable, and the sensation of heat fades over a period of fifteen to thirty minutes.

As with liquid nitrogen, some swelling and discomfort may occur at the site of the lesion, and the dead tissue will slough off. During this time, you may note some discomfort with sexual intercourse and increase or change in your normal vaginal discharge. Like liquid nitrogen, TCA works pretty well, but follow-up is needed to make sure that the lesion is really gone and that it doesn't recur later. In many instances, multiple treatments are needed, with the treatment intervals ranging between one and three weeks. So, follow-up, as always, is very important.

Staging of Vaginal Cancer

If the biopsy confirms that you have vaginal cancer, the staging process will begin to find the possible source of the cancer (if it did not originate in the vagina), or if the cancer has spread to other areas of the pelvis. (The methods for staging are covered on pages 151–156.)

Vaginal cancer includes the following stages:

Stage	What It Means
0	Also known as carcinoma in situ (a variant of severe vaginal dysplasia), this is found only on the surface layers of cells and only in the vagina. This is not really a form of vaginal cancer.
I	Cancer is found in the vagina, but has not spread beyond the vagina.
II	Cancer has spread to tissues outside of the vagina, but has not extended to the pelvic wall.
III	Cancer has spread to the wall of the pelvis. Cancer cells may also have spread to other organs and the lymph nodes in the pelvis.
IV-A	Cancer has spread into the bladder or rectum.
IV-B	Cancer has spread to other parts of the body such as the lungs.
Recurrent	The cancer has come back, in the vagina or elsewhere, after treatment.

Treatment

As with all cancers, vaginal cancer is treated by stage, type, and the patient's age and overall condition.

Stage 0

See the discussion of vaginal dysplasia earlier in this chapter.

Stage I

Squamous cell cancer treatment includes internal radiation therapy with or without external beam radiation therapy; wide local excision followed by reconstruction; and vaginectomy with or without lymph node dissection. For adenocarcinomas, surgery, total radical vaginectomy, and hysterectomy with lymph node dissection are usually needed. These treatments are described more fully later in this chapter and in chapter 7.

Construction of a new vagina (*neo-vagina* in medicalese) may be performed if feasible and if desired by the patient. If some tumor is left behind by the surgery, then additional radiation therapy should be considered. Combined local therapy may also be used, including wide local excision, lymph node sampling, and radiation therapy.

Stage II

Stage II treatment of either squamous cell or adenocarcinoma usually includes combined internal and external radiation therapy. Surgery with or without radiation therapy may also be considered.

Stage III

Treatment of either squamous cell or adenocarcinoma is the same as, but more extensive than, Stage II. Greater emphasis is placed on radiation therapy at this stage.

Stage IV-A

Treatment is the same as, but more extensive than, Stage III.

Stage IV-B

Because the cancer has spread to other parts of the body, Stage IV-B prognosis is not good; at this point, clinical trials should be strongly considered, and chemotherapy and radiation therapy may be used for palliative purposes: to decrease symptoms, not cure the disease. There is no standard choice of chemotherapy drugs at this time.

Recurrent Vaginal Cancer

If the vaginal cancer has come back, a physician may choose to perform *pelvic exenteration*: the removal of the cervix, uterus, lower colon, rectum, or bladder, depending on where the cancer has spread. Radiation and chemotherapy can be used for curative or palliative purposes, but primarily for the latter, and clinical trials are also an option for recurrent vaginal cancer.

Treatment Options for Vaginal Cancer

Radiation Therapy

Internal and external radiation therapy are covered in chapter 7.

Wide Local Excision

Wide local excision is also a fairly simple procedure for removing early-stage cancer, although it may require some reconstruction of the vagina. Using a scalpel or laser, your physician will take out the cancer and some of the tissue around it. This both removes the cancer and provides an excellent biopsy for further examination. Recovery takes about four weeks. Depending on the depth and location of the excision, a skin graft from the buttock or thigh may be necessary to repair the vagina.

Vaginectomy

Vaginectomy, or removal of the vagina, may be necessary if the cancer has spread through the vagina. In addition, if your physician fears that the cancer may have spread, he or she may perform a lymph node dissection as well. This provides a sample for biopsy and helps in the staging process.

Surgery/Hysterectomy

Surgery to cure vaginal cancer can range from wide local excision to vaginectomy to hysterectomy. If evidence shows that the cancer has spread to nearby organs such as the uterus or ovaries, your physician may choose to perform a radical hysterectomy, described on pages 157–158. This may be followed by reconstructive surgery to rebuild the vagina.

Pelvic Exenteration

Pelvic exenteration is considered a "last resort" measure, and is usually reserved for recurrent cases. Exenteration removes the vagina, cervix, uterus, rectum, lower colon, or bladder, depending on where the cancer has spread; reconstruction of the vagina, bladder, and colon are usually necessary.

Clinical Trials

Clinical trials are excellent opportunities for advanced or recurrent cancer patients to experiment with new curative and palliative therapies. See chapter 7 for details.

Self-Exams

Cancer prognosis is always directly related to the stage of cancer and the age and general health of the patient. The earlier it's caught, the better, which is why regular Pap smears are so important. You can also find changes in your body if you do regular vaginal self-exams. At first, it may seem difficult, but if you work it into your health routine—along with a monthly breast exam—you can alert your doctor to possibly cancerous changes. A detailed description of the self-exam is included in appendix B.

Risk Factors

Vaginal cancer falls into two categories: adenocarcinoma and squamous cell carcinoma. Squamous cell may be caused by HPV, while adenocarcinoma is not caused by HPV and is more common in DES daughters.

Risk Factors for Vaginal Cancer

- **Age.** Advanced stages of vaginal cancer are usually found in women over sixty, although carcinoma in situ (severe vaginal dysplasia) has become more common among young women.
- **"DES daughters."** Women whose mothers used DES to prevent miscarriages can develop a rare glassy-cell adenocarcinoma.
- **HPV infection.** Oncogenic HPV infection causes abnormalities in squamous cells that lead to some cases of vaginal cancer.
- **HIV infection.** Loss of immunity contributes to the body's inability to fight off HPV infection and abnormal cells.
- **Low socioeconomic status.** Less access to health care and preventive measures contributes to a higher rate of cancer.
- **Other genital cancers.** Women with a history of one genital cancer are more likely to develop cancer in other areas; the reasons are that cancer cells may already exist in the region, and these women probably already possess many of the risk factors.
- **Smoking.** Smoking contributes to the development of cancer.

Conclusion

Although some vaginal cancers cannot be prevented—adenocarcinoma is extremely rare and usually occurs only in DES daughters—early detection is always the best cure. Get your annual pelvic exams, get your Pap smears, don't smoke, and do a self-examination every month. It could save your life.

CHAPTER NINE

Vulvar Dysplasia and Cancer

Vulvar cancer is very rare—it accounts for only 0.6 percent of all gynecologic cancers—but can develop as a result of HPV infection. A diagram of the vulva is shown in figure 2.1. As with vaginal cancer, though, its relationship to HPV and vulvar dysplasia, or vulvar intraepithelial neoplasia (VIN), isn't as tight as those relationships in the cervix. In other words, many cases of vulvar cancer are preceded by vulvar dysplasia and are associated with HPV infection, but some aren't. The causes of the latter type of vulvar cancer remain poorly understood.

Vulva is more or less a general term that includes every outer part of the vagina, the way the term *mouth* includes your tongue, teeth, lips, and cheeks. Here's a brief description of each part of the vulva:

- **Labia majora:** Two large, fleshy lips or folds of skin. This is the part most commonly affected by vulvar cancer.

- **Labia minora:** Smaller lips that lie inside the labia majora and surround the openings to the urethra and vagina.
- **Vestibule:** Opening of the vagina.
- **Prepuce:** A fold of skin formed by the labia minora.
- **Clitoris:** A small protruding piece of tissue sensitive to stimulation.

Although all of these parts are included under the heading "vulva," and cancer can begin on any one of them, the labia is by far the most common origination of vulvar cancer.

Vulvar cancer occurs mostly in women over fifty, but has become more common in women under forty in recent years; this could be due to more widespread infection of HPV, but we don't know for sure why yet.

In women under forty, the rate of vulvar dysplasia due to HPV infection is rising. Women over fifty tend to develop the type of vulvar cancer not associated with dysplasia or HPV.

Symptoms of Vulvar Dysplasia and Vulvar Cancer

Your vulva is visible to you and is more exposed, so unlike cervical cancer, you may notice symptoms of vulvar HPV infection, dysplasia, or cancer. Constant itching, discoloration, and differences in the way your vulva looks could all indicate vulvar dysplasia or cancer. You might also experience burning, itching, and bleeding unrelated to menstruation. In addition, if you notice small, rough, white bumps on the vulva, you may have genital warts, covered in chapters 11 and 12. Most warts on the vulva contain non-oncogenic HPV types such as 6 or 11, and these put you at little or no risk for cancer.

However—and it's a *big* however—they also indicate that you may be at increased risk for having HPV infection in other parts of the anogenital tract, with the possibility of having oncogenic HPV types. Remember, sexually transmitted agents like to travel in packs, and so do different HPV types.

Diagnosis of Vulvar Dysplasia

A regular pelvic exam is the best defense against vulvar dysplasia and vulvar cancer. Although Pap smears are useful to detect cervical and vaginal dysplasia, they're not particularly helpful to diagnose vulvar dysplasia, since it's found on the external genitals. If your doctor suspects vulvar dysplasia, you'll probably be asked to come in for a colposcopy. This is a good idea anyway, since as I said earlier, if you have vulvar lesions, you're at increased risk of having cervical, vaginal, or anal lesions.

The process for colposcopic examination is much the same for the vulva as it is for the cervix and vagina, and the biopsy will be examined by a pathologist. The doctor usually numbs the suspicious area with a lidocaine injection. He or she then uses biopsy forceps (similar to those used for cervical biopsies) to obtain a sample of vulvar tissue. As with a vaginal biopsy, you may notice some bleeding and some discomfort once the anesthetic wears off. Healing will probably take several days, and you'll be expected to keep the area dry and clean to prevent infection. If your biopsy shows cancerous changes, then you'll have to go through staging as described on pages 151–156. If it shows vulvar dysplasia, then you'll be treated as described below.

Staging and Treatment of Vulvar Dysplasia

If the biopsy shows that you have vulvar dysplasia, then by definition you don't have cancer. As in the cervix and vagina, vulvar disease is staged as mild, moderate, or severe dysplasia—VIN 1, VIN 2, or VIN 3, respectively. The same criteria are used to stage the lesions as those in the cervix and vagina. As in the cervix and vagina, moderate and severe lesions need to be removed, and mild cases can be treated or watched carefully to make sure they go away on their own.

The treatment of vulvar dysplasia is based on the same principles as those for cervical and vaginal disease: removal of the affected tissues. In the vulva, several methods can remove the lesions, and the choice depends on a number of factors, including the size of the lesion, its location, and the experience and preferences of your doctor.

Generally, to treat vulvar dysplasia, the usual approaches are wide local excision or laser therapy. Your doctor may try 5 percent fluorouracil cream as well, but it has a lower response rate of 50 to 60 percent. Liquid nitrogen or TCA may occasionally be used for mild vulvar dysplasia. Sometimes the lesion requires a *skinning vulvectomy*, a procedure that is described in greater detail later in this chapter.

Staging of Vulvar Cancer

The following stages are used for vulvar cancer:

Stage	What It Means
0	Also known as carcinoma in situ (a variant of severe vulvar dysplasia), this is found only on the surface of the skin on the vulva. This isn't really a form of vulvar cancer.
I	Cancer is found only in the vulva and/or the perineum (the space between the opening of the rectum and vagina). The tumor is less than 2 cm in size.
II	Cancer is found in the perineum and the tumor is larger than 2 cm in size.
III	Cancer in the vulva and/or perineum and has spread to nearby tissues such as the lower part of the urethra, vagina, anus, and nearby lymph nodes.
IV	Cancer has spread beyond the immediate area and into the lining of the bladder or rectum. It also may have spread to the lymph nodes or other parts of the body.
Recurrent	The cancer has come back, in the vulva or elsewhere, after treatment.

Survival rates for vulvar cancer are good, but in keeping with the themes presented throughout this book, the earlier the cancer is caught, the better your prognosis.

Treatment

As with all cancers, treatment depends on the stage of cancer, your age, and your overall condition. Surgery is the most common treatment, with radiation and chemotherapy being used only in the more advanced stages.

Stage 0

This is equivalent to vulvar carcinoma in situ, or severe dysplasia. It's not cancer, and is treated as described in the section on vulvar dysplasia.

Stage I

Again, wide local excision is effective, but because the cancer has spread below the skin's surface, your physician may choose one of the following: radical local excision and groin lymph node removal; radical vulvectomy and groin lymph node removal; or, in selected patients, radiation only. Lymph nodes are removed to diagnose the presence of cancer. Those treatments are described more fully later in this chapter.

Stage II

Since the cancer has spread to the perineum, radical vulvectomy with removal of the lymph nodes in the groin in both sides of the body is necessary. If cancer cells are found in the lymph nodes, radiation may be given to the pelvis. In selected patients—those who cannot undergo surgery for health reasons—radiation therapy alone may be used.

Stage III

In Stage III vulvar cancer, the disease has spread to the surrounding tissues and organs. Radical vulvectomy and removal of the lymph nodes—both in the groin and upper part of the thigh on both sides of the body—is the most effective treatment. If cancer cells are found in the lymph nodes, radiation to the pelvis and groin could kill any remaining cells. If the tumor has spread throughout the area, radiation and chemotherapy could be used, followed by radical vulvectomy and removal of lymph nodes on both sides of the body. Again, in selected patients, radiation—with or without chemotherapy—is also an option.

Stage IV

Depending on where the cancer has spread, radical vulvectomy and pelvic exenteration (removal of the lower colon, rectum, bladder, uterus, cervix, and vagina) may remove the cancerous cells. Other options include radical vulvectomy followed by radiation therapy; radiation therapy followed by radical vulvectomy; radiation therapy with or without chemotherapy, and with or without surgery.

Recurrent Vulvar Cancer

Wide local excision or a radical vulvectomy and pelvic exenteration are both options for patients who haven't previously had these procedures. Other treatments include radiation therapy plus chemotherapy, with or without surgery; palliative (symptom-reducing, but not curative) radiation therapy; and experimental treatments being tested in clinical trials.

Treatment Options for Vulvar Cancer

Wide Local Excision

Wide local excision removes the part of the vulva affected by the cancer and some of the surrounding skin, and is a common treatment for isolated cancerous lesions. Using a "cold-knife" method or laser, this operation can be done in a hospital or as an outpatient procedure. Because of the sensitivity of the area, healing may take several weeks to a month. Chapter 6 covers several outpatient procedures, such as LEEP for dysplasia, and the procedure is much the same. The primary difference is that infection is a much more pressing concern, since the excision is done on the outside of the body. Follow your doctor's orders as closely as possible with concern to showering, sexual intercourse, lifting heavy objects, and general care for the excised area.

Skinning Vulvectomy

As unpleasant as the name is, a skinning vulvectomy is an excellent treatment for early-stage vulvar cancer and dysplasia. It removes the epidermis and dermis (the skin) of the vulva to retain both cosmetic and functional use. The procedure is fairly lengthy, meticulous, and requires a highly skilled surgeon. In addition, you'll need to stay in a hospital for several days to heal. The primary benefits of skinning vulvectomy are that (1) it provides an excellent sample for pathologic examination to determine if the cancer has become invasive; and (2) the cosmetic and functional results are excellent.

Radical Local Excision with Groin Lymph Node Dissection

Radical local excision, like wide local excision, removes the cancer as well as the surrounding area. Removing the lymph nodes provides a biopsy to find out if the cancer has spread. Because lymph node dissection requires surgery, this procedure will require a few days' hospital stay.

Radiation Therapy

External radiation therapy is covered in detail in chapter 7.

Radical Vulvectomy with Lymph Node Dissection

The radical vulvectomy used to be the standard treatment for vulvar cancer, but an increasing trend toward conservatism—doing as little surgery as possible—has made this surgery less common. Radical vulvectomy removes the entire vulva, including the labia, clitoris, and prepuce. Surgery usually follows a radical vulvectomy to reconstruct the labia and retain some cosmetic and functional value. Both are major surgeries and require a hospital stay. The "subtotal" vulvectomy does not remove the entire vulva, and can be an alternative to radical vulvectomy.

Pelvic Exenteration

Pelvic exenteration includes the removal of all internal organs in the pelvis: the vulva, vagina, uterus, ovaries, and possibly part of the colon as well. The extensive surgery requires a long hospital stay and reconstructive surgery for diverting urine flow and possibly a colostomy (the surgical creation of a hole through which waste can pass). It's considered a last resort and is only used when the cancer has metastasized throughout the pelvis.

Clinical Trials

Clinical trials are excellent opportunities for advanced or recurrent cancer patients to experiment with new curative and palliative therapies. See chapter 7 for details.

Self-Examination

The prognosis for cancer patients is always best when the cancer is caught early. Regular pelvic examinations help your physician catch any early abnormalities, but you can help yourself on a monthly basis by performing regular self-examinations. The procedure for doing a vulvar exam is fairly simple and it's outlined in appendix B.

Risk Factors for Vulvar Cancer

The risks attached to vulvar cancer are similar to cervical cancer, but warrant repeating. Keep in mind that *all* risk factors involved with HPV infection—multiple partners, intercourse with an infected partner, unprotected intercourse—are also risk factors for vulvar cancer.

Risk Factors for Vulvar Cancer

- **Age.** Seventy-five percent of women with vulvar cancer are over age fifty, and 66 percent are over seventy.
- **Chronic vulvar inflammation.**
- **HPV infection.** Although HPV is not a direct cause every time, about 50 percent of vulvar cancers are directly linked to HPV infection.
- **HIV infection.** Loss of immunity contributes to the body's inability to fight off HPV infection and abnormal cells.
- **Lichen sclerosis,** a condition occurring mostly in postmenopausal women that can cause severe itchiness in the vulva and may increase the chance of malignancy.
- **Low socioeconomic status.** As with cervical cancer, less access to health care and preventive measures contributes to a higher rate of cancer.
- **Other genital cancers.** Women with a history of one genital cancer are more likely to develop cancer in other areas; the reasons are that cancer cells may already exist in the region, and these women probably already possess many of the risk factors.
- **Smoking.** Smoking increases the risk of developing cancer. Stop smoking, if possible.

Conclusion

While vulvar cancer is quite rare, the incidences of both vulvar dysplasia and cancer have increased recently. Because many cases of vulvar dysplasia are attributed to HPV infection, more young women are being diagnosed with and treated for these precancerous lesions. In addition, because of the increasing age of the population, more older women are developing vulvar cancer. As with all HPV-related cancers, vigilance and prevention are the best medicines.

CHAPTER TEN

Anal Dysplasia and Cancer

You may be surprised to find a chapter devoted to anal cancer and its precursors in this book. Anal cancer is *not* on most people's radar screens. Granted, most of the subject matter of this book isn't exactly idle chitchat, but you can imagine that anal cancer and anal HPV infection top the "I don't want to talk about it" list in that category! Basically, any discussion of the anus and its various functions and diseases is taboo in our society. We don't talk much publicly about sex, we don't hear much about HPV or genital warts or cervical cancer, and we *certainly* don't talk about those things as they relate to anal cancer. Above all, as a society we don't acknowledge the anus as a sexual organ, and this prevents us from acknowledging the complications that can arise from using it in this way.

The notion of anal sex carries all sorts of baggage. Many people associate homosexuality with receptive anal intercourse, and it is, in fact, one of the sex acts in the repertoire of many men who have sex with men (Men who have Sex with Men: MSM to researchers). What you may not realize is that a remarkably high proportion of sexually active women in our society practice *heterosexual* anal intercourse. In this context, anal intercourse occurs when a man's penis is inserted into a woman's anal canal. Accurate numbers are tough to come by, but depending on which survey you read, between 20 percent and 45 percent (and possibly even more) of all American women have anal intercourse at least once in their lives. This means that of all the people in this country who have had anal intercourse, the majority are heterosexual women!

Why do people practice anal intercourse? We know what the main function of the anus is: It primarily acts as a transit area for fecal matter as it passes from the rectum to the outside of our bodies. Although the anal sphincters play a major role in holding feces in and preventing incontinence, few people realize that the anus doesn't actually hold fecal matter for any appreciable period of time—the rectum is the real holding area.

In fact, the anus plays another role: It's a sexual organ just like the other members of the genital club. The area around the outside part of the anus (the *perianal area* in medicalese) is extremely sensitive to touch. Although insertion of objects such as a penis, a finger, or toys can hurt, the sensation of these objects inside the anal canal is also pleasurable for some. In men, some of this pleasure is derived from having objects rub against their prostate gland.

Besides the sexual pleasure involved in anal intercourse, some women have other reasons to engage in anal sex. For obvious reasons, anal sex won't lead to pregnancy.

Younger women may choose to have anal intercourse because they believe it preserves their virginity. Finally, because of all the taboo and emotional baggage attached to anal intercourse, having anal intercourse with a woman may be a form of domination for some men. Regardless of the reason, all of the sexually transmitted agents that can infect the cervix can also infect the anal canal. Unfortunately, that means HPV, too.

Before we get to anal HPV and anal cancer, I'd like to make just a few more points. First, any items inserted into the anal canal could also spread infections. HPV could spread to the anal canal of a woman through insertion of a penis that has a lesion on it. HPV might also be spread through insertion of fingers or toys such as dildos or vibrators.

Second, it's possible to get anal HPV infection even if nothing has ever been inserted into your anal canal. If you have HPV infection in the cervix, vulva, or vagina, cells shed into the vaginal fluids might carry infectious HPV with them. The material could spread to the perianal region and then into the opening of the anus.

Likewise, material can spread from the anus to the cervix. How do we know this? Most urinary tract infections are due to fecal bacteria such as *E. coli*. This could be due to the way some women wipe themselves after a bowel movement. (Some doctors recommend that a women wipe from front to back, not back to front.) Basically, we're not sure *how* stuff really gets around; we just know that it *does*. Based on everything you now know, you shouldn't be surprised to hear that women with cervical cancer are at higher risk of anal cancer than the general population of women, and women with anal cancer are at higher risk of cervical cancer than the general population of women. The same goes for the relationship between vulvar and anal disease, and probably for vaginal and anal disease as well.

So why am I telling you all this? Anal cancer is more common among women than among men in our society (although the risk is highest among MSM, in whom the incidence of anal cancer is about as high as cervical cancer was in women before we instituted cervical Pap smear screening). It's also because the incidence of anal cancer continues to rise every year among women. In the United States, we estimate that the incidence of anal cancer is about 0.9 per 100,000 women, roughly one-tenth that of the current incidence of cervical cancer. Finally, the incidence of anal cancer is estimated to be about seven times higher among women at especially high risk, such as HIV-positive women. Roughly 2,000 women will be diagnosed with anal cancer this year. This isn't a big number—roughly the same incidence as vulvar cancer and about half the incidence of vaginal cancer—but as I said, the numbers are growing every year. The reasons for this growth aren't clear, but perhaps it reflects changes in sexual practices in the last few decades. With changes in attitudes toward sex, I'm guessing that anal intercourse may have been practiced more commonly among women in the last few decades, and this has increased their risk of acquiring anal HPV infection.

Since it probably takes many years from the time of initial anal HPV infection to the development of anal cancer, this increase is only beginning to show up in the last few years. If this is true, then the incidence of anal cancer will continue to grow even further in the future. And of course, nobody screens for anal cancer the way we screen for cervical cancer.

Anal HPV Infection

Physiologically, the anus and cervix have a lot in common, so it's no wonder that the anus is also susceptible to HPV infection. Like the cervix, the anus has a transformation zone (TZ), shown in figure 10.1.

In the cervix, as you know, the TZ is where the columnar cells of the endocervical canal meet the squamous cells of the exocervix. In the anal canal, the transformation zone is where the columnar epithelium of the rectum meets the squamous epithelium of the anus. This anorectal junction is not visible on the outside, but occurs 2 to 4 centimeters inside the anal canal. As in the cervix, HPV likes to infect the anal transformation zone. This is also, not surprisingly, where most of the anal cancers and precancerous anal lesions arise.

Now we come to the obligatory discussion of terminology: As in the cervix, vulva, and vagina, anal disease is staged as anal intraepithelial neoplasia (AIN), which can be classified as mild anal dysplasia, moderate anal dysplasia, or severe anal dysplasia: AIN 1, AIN 2, and AIN 3. The same criteria are used to stage the lesions in the anus as those in the cervix, vagina, and vulva. As in the cervix, vagina, and vulva, moderate and severe anal lesions need to be removed, and mild anal dysplasia could be treated or watched carefully to make sure it goes away on its own.

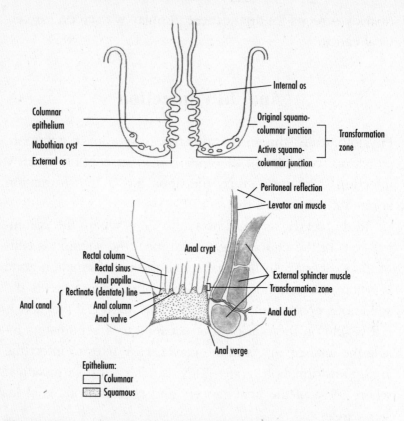

Figure 10.1: Comparison of the Transformation Zone of the Cervix to the Anus. *This diagram compares the cervical transformation zone (TZ) of the cervix to that of the anus. The TZ of the anus is not visible on routine perianal examination. In the cervix (upper panel) the TZ is where the columnar epithelium of the endocervical canal meets the squamous epithelium of the exocervix. In the anus, shown in the bottom panel, the TZ is where the columnar epithelium of the rectum meets the squamous epithelium of the anus. (Illustration by Ira C. Smith.)*

And like HPV infection anywhere on the body, anal HPV infection can be found in the absence of any disease at all.

What do we know about anal HPV infection in women? We really don't know much about what is going on in healthy women in the general population. We do have a growing body of knowledge about women at increased risk of anal HPV infection because they're either HIV-positive or they practice high-risk sexual behaviors—commercial sex workers or women who use intravenous drugs. These data are surprising: So far, in each study, the prevalence of anal HPV infection is higher in both of these groups than is cervical HPV infection! If one looks at the HPV types in the anal canal, they tend to be the same types as those found in the cervix.

As I said, we don't know as much about healthy, average women, but I suspect that anal HPV infection isn't nearly as common as in these high-risk women. It's probably not as common as cervical HPV infection in the general population. Nevertheless, women are indeed at risk of having anal HPV infection.

As I implied earlier, exactly how you get anal HPV is unknown, but receptive anal sex is probably the best way. Having said that, other ways are certainly possible as well, and these include inserting objects or fingers into the anal canal. In addition, perianal infection—HPV infection in the area outside the opening of the anus—can probably be acquired by scratching or touching an HPV-infected area on yourself or your sexual partner, and then scratching or touching your own perianal area. And don't forget shaving!

Anal Dysplasia

As you might guess, if HPV can infect the anal canal, it can cause lesions there, the same way it does in the cervix. Just as we have little information on anal HPV infection in the general population of women, we have little information on anal dysplasia in women. Once again, it's probably reasonable to guess that it's quite uncommon, given the relative rarity of anal cancer in this group. Conversely, we do know that anal dysplasia is common among high-risk women. This is *not* a surprise, given the high prevalence of anal HPV infection in these women.

Symptoms of Anal Dysplasia

Dysplasia inside the anal canal is not usually visible, but sometimes becomes apparent when a woman notices new bleeding with bowel movements or blood on the toilet paper after a bowel movement. This can be a sign of warts or anal dysplasia in the anal canal. (Bleeding can also be a sign of cancer in the colon or rectum, so be sure to tell your doctor immediately.) Occasionally, a lesion becomes apparent if it grows big enough to protrude through the anal canal to the outside. Developing pain can indicate anal cancer—anal warts and dysplasia are usually painless.

Anal dysplasia in the perianal area is usually more obvious, since you can see and feel it. A picture of one such lesion is shown in figure 10.2. A dark discoloration may be noted, or you may feel a bump. The area may itch or bleed, particularly after a bowel movement.

If you experience any of these symptoms, you should

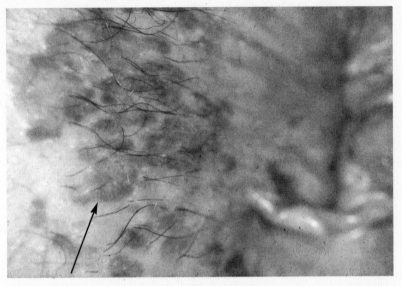

Figure 10.2: Bowen's Disease. *This figure shows a picture of Bowen's Disease, which occurs on the area outside of the opening of the anus. It is typically colored more darkly (see arrow) than surrounding normal tissue and on biopsy shows severe dysplasia. It has the potential to progress to anal cancer if not treated. (Author's photo.)*

see your doctor immediately. Subclinical infection, the kind more often inside the anal canal, though, exhibits no outward symptoms, and can be detected only through screening procedures.

Who Should Be Screened?

At the moment, screening in the anal canal (as we strongly recommend in the cervix) is not widely performed, and it's not considered the "standard of care." Why? Several reasons.

One: We don't have direct evidence that anal dysplasia is the precursor lesion to anal cancer in the same way that cervical dysplasia is the precursor to cervical cancer. Having said that, the main reason is simply that we haven't looked, and all indications are that anal dysplasia is, indeed, an anal cancer precursor. Two: While the risk is clear in some of the high-risk groups mentioned previously, the risk in the general population of healthy women is not known but is probably quite a bit lower. No one really knows if the incidence of anal cancer is high enough in the general population to merit routine screening of healthy women; my guess is that it probably isn't. Three: Since all of this information is quite new, many doctors simply aren't aware of it.

So—who *do* I recommend for screening? For now, I've been careful to make formal recommendations only for MSM, for whom we have the most data. The data we've collected so far on women suggest that three groups should be considered for screening, outlined below.

Who Should Be Considered for Anal Pap Smear Screening

- HIV-positive women.
- Women at high risk because of commercial sex work or use of intravenous drugs.
- Women with a history of multiple anal receptive intercourse partners.
- Women with a history of perianal warts.
- Women with a history of vaginal or vulvar dysplasia. (It's also possible that women with a history of cervical dysplasia are at risk.)
- Women with a history of cancer at any of these sites should be considered for anal screening, since there's evidence of increased risk among women with those diagnoses.

This is my *personal* opinion, and you won't find these recommendations listed formally by any medical organization.

Having an Anal Pap Smear

So now you've read this list and think you should ask your doctor to be screened for anal disease. How is it done? Because of the many similarities between the anus and the cervix, the anal canal lends itself quite well to anal Pap smear screening. The anal canal is moist, and an anal swab inserted into the anal canal can collect cells just like a cervical cytobrush collects cervical cells. I strongly recommend that the doctor use a special kind of swab called a Dacron swab and that it be moistened in tap water before being inserted into the anal canal. A photo of an anal Pap smear is shown in figure 10.3.

However, because so little is known at this point, anal Pap smear screening is not done routinely. It's been used in several research studies of high-risk individuals such as MSM, HIV-positive men and women, and commercial sex workers. If you ask about having one done, your doctor will probably look at you like you're crazy, since many haven't even heard of it. But you can refer them to this book and to the growing body of literature that supports its use in high-risk women.

Having an anal Pap smear is uncomfortable but by no means terrible; it mostly just feels weird. After the swab has been used to collect the cells, the doctor will either smear the cells on a glass slide just as they would with a cervical Pap smear, or they can use the ThinPrep method. (In fact,

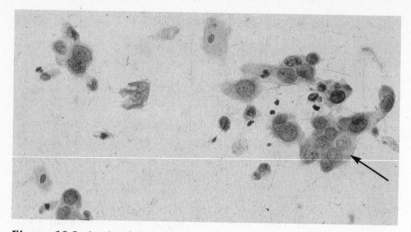

Figure 10.3: An Anal Pap Smear. *This photo shows cells collected from an anal Pap smear. The arrow shows cells consistent with severe anal dysplasia. Overall, anal Pap smears closely resemble cervical Pap smears. (Photo courtesy of Dr. Teresa Darragh, University of California, San Francisco.)*

I recommend the latter because it's a little easier to use if your doctor has only limited experience in performing anal Pap smears.)

Often, the doctor is afraid to hurt you, and so he or she doesn't push the swab in far enough. I recommend pushing it in as far as it will go—it won't get "lost" because it always hits the wall of the rectum and stops there. The doctor also needs to twirl the swab on the way out to increase the number of cells collected. One last word of caution: You might be tempted to perform an anal douche or enema, thinking that you are helping the doctor. In fact, fecal matter rarely gets in the way of the test, and when you douche or have an enema, you are effectively rinsing away the cells that would be of most interest to the cytotechnologist.

The cells are sent to the cytotechnologist or cytopathologist for interpretation, and I recommend using the same Bethesda criteria that are used for interpretation of cervical Pap smears. The various levels of anal lesions can therefore be divided into normal, ASCUS, anal LSIL, or anal HSIL. As in the cervix, anal HSIL probably poses the biggest cancer threat.

How often should you have an anal Pap smear if your first one is normal? This is a question that hasn't yet been answered with any kind of data, so I'm winging this one. Remember, just as in the cervix, anal Pap smears are far from perfect, so *repeated* Pap smears might be needed to identify anal dysplasia before it can progress to cancer. If you are an HIV-negative woman at high risk, and you continue to have these risks, then you should consider having an anal Pap smear every two to three years. Anal cancer develops slowly, so intervals of two to three years between repeat anal Pap smears should suffice for HIV-negative patients. If your risk factors go away, then you could have them less often, such as every five years. If you're an HIV-positive woman, you should probably have an anal Pap annually.

What Happens When One of Your Anal Paps Comes Back Abnormal?

Basically, I recommend that any woman with an abnormal anal Pap smear, including ASCUS, should be sent for further evaluation.

Just as in the cervix, the next step in the evaluation of a woman with an abnormal anal Pap smear is to visualize and biopsy the lesions. The procedure actually uses a cervical colposcope, but to distinguish it from cervical colposcopy, I call the procedure *high-resolution anoscopy*, or HRA for short. The procedure is modeled on cervical colposcopy and uses all the same tricks: magnification, vinegar, Lugol's solution—the works.

Getting an HRA is one of the trickier parts of the evaluation, since relatively few individuals in the country are trained in this procedure at this point. However, my group continues to train more and more people, and right now you should be able to find a qualified doctor in most major American cities. Sorting out the insurance issues and payment is another story, since many insurers don't yet cover this procedure.

High-Resolution Anoscopy

The first part of the examination should include feeling the groin for evidence of lymph node swelling, since this can indicate spread of anal cancer. Next, the doctor should inspect the perianal region for signs of warts or anal dysplasia. Then comes a digital exam—digital in the old-fashioned sense, not the computer sense! During a digital examination, wearing thin gloves, your doctor will feel the outside of the anus for any lumps, unusual redness, swelling, or irritation. Then he or she will put a lubricated finger into the rectum and gently feel for lumps. This may cause you some discomfort. He or she may also check the glove for evidence of blood.

After the digital examination, the doctor will perform HRA.

First, the doctor inserts a small disposable plastic

anoscope to allow the placement of a stick wrapped with a gauze pad soaked in acetic acid. Note that in the cervix we use 5 percent acetic acid—regular old vinegar. In the anal canal we dilute it some, since it's a little too irritating, and use it as a 3 percent solution. After removing the anoscope, the acetic-acid–soaked gauze-wrapped stick remains in place for at least one minute to allow absorption of the acetic acid by the anal mucosa.

Then your doctor removes the stick, reinserts the anoscope, and performs an examination of the aceto-whitened lesions with the help of a colposcope. The doctor slowly withdraws the anoscope as he or she completes the examination, and this part of the examination is modestly uncomfortable. Having the anoscope in gives you a feeling of pressure and makes you feel like you want to have a bowel movement. Don't worry, though—you won't! The acetic acid itself can be somewhat uncomfortable, since it feels quite cold and can sting, particularly if you're experiencing anal irritation for any reason.

With HRA the appearance of anal and cervical lesions is similar; they each become whiter with more advanced disease, and the "mosaic" or "coarse" vascular patterns of the lesions are alike, as well. A picture of an anal lesion seen through the colposcope during an HRA procedure is shown in figure 10.4. Your doctor will take a biopsy of the most severe-looking lesions using small biopsy forceps—considerably smaller than those used for the cervix. The higher up you go into the anal canal, the fewer the number of nerve endings; you won't need any kind of an anesthetic for an anal biopsy if it's near the transformation zone. In fact, for most biopsies taken from the anal canal, no anesthetic is necessary. You'll feel little or no pain with the biopsy, but possibly a tugging sensation. On the other hand, biopsies from the perianal area do require an anesthetic—typically an injection into the lesion with 1 percent lidocaine to numb it. Afterward, you may experience some anal pain and bleeding as the biopsy site heals. The bottom line (pardon the pun): Anal biopsies are not nearly as bad as you might think.

ASCUS or LSIL on an anal Pap smear can represent moderate or severe anal dysplasia in disguise, just as in the cervix, which is why I recommend HRA for all patients with any anal abnormalities. Once the anal biopsy is done, the tissue is dropped into a formalin jar and processed the same way as cervical biopsies. Interpretation of the severity of anal disease entails the same criteria as for cervical disease. You may also request the Hybrid Capture II test (I mentioned this earlier; it tests for the presence of HPV DNA) to help you and your doctor decide the best route for treatment, but at this point, we haven't determined the best use of this test in the anal canal.

Treatment of Anal Dysplasia

The treatment issues for anal dysplasia are similar to those we have already discussed for cervical, vaginal, and vulvar dysplasia. Moderate and severe anal dysplasia should probably be treated, and mild cases could be followed. On the other hand, many women prefer having the lesions removed from the anal canal, regardless of whether they are mild, moderate, or severe anal dysplasia. Unfortunately, treatment of lesions in the anal canal is more diffi-

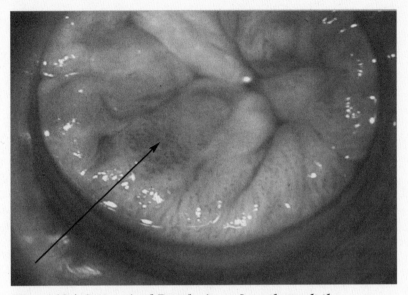

**Figure 10.4: Severe Anal Dysplasia as Seen through the
Colposcope.** *This photo shows the appearance of severe anal dysplasia
seen through the colposcope after application of 3 percent acetic acid
(see arrow). Like severe cervical dysplasia, severe anal dysplasia is flat,
turns white with the acetic acid, and has an abnormal blood vessel
pattern. This one shows a pattern called "punctation." Lesions like this
would normally be missed on routine anoscopic inspection of the anal
canal and only become visible with acetic acid and magnification.
(Author's photo.)*

cult than those of the cervix. In the cervix, LEEP easily removes the entire cervical transformation zone, with relatively few long-term consequences. In the anal canal,
removal of the entire anal TZ is impossible. Remember that
the anal canal is essentially a tube and that the TZ is like a
band of that tube—it goes around the entire circumference
of the tube where the anus meets the rectum.

For surgical treatment of anal dysplasia in a day-surgery
type of setting, the main complication is pain. Surgery is

resorted to when the lesions are too large to be treated with application of liquid nitrogen, TCA, or special creams. The surgical treatment procedures themselves don't hurt much, since you'll have some form of anesthesia. But after the anesthesia wears off, watch out!

On the other hand, if you're being treated with application of TCA or liquid nitrogen, the pain factor is not nearly as bad. More on that later. Another complication of treatment of very large anal lesions is stenosis, which basically means scarring that causes the diameter of the tube to narrow and leads to difficulties in having bowel movements. This happens very rarely, but probably results from trying to remove too much of that circumferential transition zone. On the other end of the spectrum, if the anal sphincters are damaged during therapy, anal incontinence, or the ability to hold in a bowel movement, may result. Again, these problems are exceedingly rare. Other very rare complications are abscesses or infections in the anal canal and excessive anal bleeding.

So how is the treatment of AIN dysplasia approached? If you have mild anal dysplasia, you may opt simply to have it followed with a repeat HRA every three to four months.

If the lesion doesn't regress on its own, then you may consider therapy. Here, we divide the lesions into intra-anal—lesions *inside* the anus—and perianal—lesions *around* the anus—since the treatment approaches are different.

Treatment of Mild Anal Dysplasia

For intra-anal lesions, if the lesions are relatively small and limited in number, treatment can usually be done in the office, with application of TCA or liquid nitrogen. Neither of these methods require any anesthesia, and both may require multiple follow-up visits and re-treatment to ensure that the lesions really go away. After the treatments, you may experience some mild anal discomfort, minor bleeding, and possibly some discharge. In the unlikely event that you notice a lot of bleeding, severe pain, or swelling, notify your doctor immediately.

A new approach is called infrared coagulation (IRC). Already approved for the treatment of hemorrhoids, with IRC the doctor places a probe on the surface of the lesion and delivers a pulse of infrared energy. This essentially bakes the tissue and kills the abnormal cells. Trials are planned to determine this method's effectiveness for different grades of anal dysplasia.

On the other hand, if the internal lesions are too large, the methods described above probably won't work. In this case, if you choose to have therapy, the only alternative is anal surgery, described below. After any of these treatments, you'll need periodic assessment with anal Pap smears and HRA to make sure that the lesions do not recur.

More treatment options for perianal disease are discussed in chapter 12, "Methods of Treatment for Genital Warts."

Treatment of Moderate and Severe Anal Dysplasia

If the moderate or severe anal dysplasia is *inside* your anus (intra-anal), you should probably get it treated if you can. The same considerations apply as if you have mild anal dysplasia—if the lesions are small enough, they can probably be treated in the office with TCA or liquid nitrogen. If they're too large, anal surgery may be necessary.

If you have moderate or severe anal dysplasia around your anus (perianal), then once again, the treatment varies depending on the extent of the lesion. Some of these lesions are also called Bowen's disease (see fig. 10.2). Smaller lesions can be treated with TCA or liquid nitrogen. Bigger lesions may be treated with laser therapy. Lesions that surround the entire anal opening may have to be treated with a more aggressive surgical procedure.

After all is said and done, a patient may choose to put off treatment and opt for close follow-up. This isn't necessarily a bad choice. Some patients have such widespread lesions that the chances of clearing them are small, and the risks involved in undergoing the treatments are large. Even if the lesions are potentially treatable, given the pain of anal surgery and the uncertainty that it will help to prevent cancer, following the lesions without treatment might be a good choice. After all, the odds are still in your favor—only a small percentage of patients will progress to invasive cancer (the exact number is not known but it's probably less than 5 percent), and the likelihood is that the anal dysplasia will not progress to cancer for many years, if at all.

On the other hand, no one can predict who will develop anal cancer, and it could be fatal if you're one of the unlucky ones. My personal opinion is that these lesions should be treated whenever possible. But when one of my patients is reluctant to have surgery, I support them in their decision . . . *as long as they agree to return for regular follow-up.* If a patient has severe anal dysplasia, I usually see them every three to four months and repeat the HRA, looking for clinical signs of progression to invasive cancer. I also tell them to contact me right away if they notice any warning signs of cancer: pain, new bleeding, swelling in their groin lymph nodes, or rapid growth of a new lesion.

If I have a high-risk patient who I know *a priori* is a poor surgical candidate, I still believe that it's worthwhile to do an anal Pap smear and HRA, even if I know that they won't undergo treatment if they're diagnosed with severe anal dysplasia. Why? Because at least I *know* they're at risk of progressing to anal cancer. I *know* this is someone to watch every three to four months, because the earlier a cancer is detected and treated, the better the outcome. If they were never screened in the first place, chances are that if they develop cancer, they won't seek medical attention until the cancer is more advanced and the chances for successful treatment are lower.

Finally, if we begin to perform anal Pap smear screening on high-risk women on a more routine basis, treatment will be much easier in these women. Why? Because if we're more proactive about identifying anal dysplasia in women even before they become symptomatic, chances are that the lesions will be detected when they're at an earlier, smaller stage. Remember that if the lesions are sufficiently small, they can often be treated quite easily with TCA and liquid nitrogen. Surgery may not be necessary. So if we start to screen women routinely, more and more of the lesions will probably be found at the stage where the treatment should be pretty straightforward and minimally uncomfortable.

As it is right now, in the absence of screening, we only see women whose lesions have advanced to the point where they have developed some of these symptoms. Treating these women is much harder than treating women in the earlier stages of the disease. So this is clearly an issue that the medical community needs to discuss, and as a medical consumer, you should make your voice heard, too.

Treatment Options for Moderate and Severe Anal Dysplasia

Research on the treatment of moderate and severe anal dysplasia is still in its early stages, but the available options include surgical excision with electrocautery or scalpel; laser; liquid nitrogen; and application of local therapies such as trichloroacetic (TCA) or bichoroacetic acid.

Surgical Excision

Similar to the LEEP and cold-knife conization methods of cervical treatments, surgical excision is a method for both removing the lesion and providing a biopsy for further study. Excision can often be done as an outpatient procedure, and is usually reserved for patients whose lesions are too big to treat with TCA or liquid nitrogen. This procedure is also used to biopsy patients more widely if there's concern about anal cancer. The biopsy procedures I discussed earlier in this chapter are well tolerated because they're pretty limited. If I feel that a patient needs lots of biopsies or biopsies that are deeper than what I can comfortably do in the office, then I refer them to the anal surgeon for surgical excision.

One important point to note: The anal surgeon who does the procedure must be familiar with using HRA, magnification, and acetic acid. Most surgeons were not trained to use these procedures—they use standard anoscopes without magnification. This allows them to easily see and treat the bumpy lesions. Unfortunately, those are more likely to be low-grade lesions, the kind that are really annoying, but which won't kill you. The high-grade lesions such as moderate and severe anal dysplasia, on the other hand, will often be missed entirely unless the surgeon uses vinegar and magnification. In my opinion, one of the worst things that could happen is that a woman undergoes the entire surgical procedure without having adequate treatment of the areas of greatest concern.

On the day of the surgery, you'll go to the surgery center, where the staff will insert an intravenous line, give you a sedative, and take you to the operating room. You'll be given a light general anesthetic or occasionally a spinal anesthetic, or even a local block.

The surgeon will insert an instrument called a retractor, which will spread open the anal canal to allow easier access. The surgeon will insert the vinegar and examine the whole area under magnification. He or she will then biopsy widely. Lesions that remain after the biopsying is done are removed with a scalpel or destroyed with electrocautery, the use of an electric current to destroy the tissues. The whole procedure usually takes less than an hour. You'll be packed with gauze and sent to the recovery room to wake up.

You'll usually be allowed to go home later in the day, and here's where the hard part begins. Postoperative pain can be *really* bad—I've heard some patients describing it as a 20 on a scale of 1 to 10. The pain can be constant or it may occur primarily with bowel movements. Sometimes, it's bad enough to lay you up for as much as three weeks, so I usually recommend that you plan to take some time off if you're going to have this procedure.

Having said all of this awful stuff, I'd like you to know that the surgeons *are* getting better at pain control. You'll likely be sent home with some nonnarcotic pain medications and possibly some narcotics for short-term pain control. Muscle relaxants such as members of the Valium family (*benzodiazepines* in medicalese) can help. A cream that appears to be very useful is called Elamax-5, and it contains lidocaine to help dull the pain. Sitz baths (in which you sit in a tub of lukewarm salted water) and other ointments such as zinc oxide can also be soothing and promote healing.

Other than pain, the possible major complications of the surgery include stenosis if too much tissue is removed, incontinence if the anal sphincter muscles are damaged, abscess or infection, and bleeding. However, these complications are quite rare.

At this point, we don't have a lot of data regarding the effectiveness of any of these treatments, including surgery, to prevent recurrence of moderate or severe anal dysplasia, and we don't know how effective they are at preventing development of anal cancer. Nevertheless, it would take many thousands of patients and up to several decades to collect that information, and if it were me, I don't think I would want to wait to find out how that experiment turned out. So, some of the information I've given you isn't really based on data, but on common sense (at least my idea of common sense).

Laser

Laser ablation uses a laser to simultaneously remove and cauterize the lesion, and is a fairly quick procedure. Basically, it's similar to the cold-knife excision, except that a laser is used to destroy the tissue instead of removing it or destroying it with electricity. Laser ablation is sometimes done in a surgeon's office instead of a day-surgery center. As for complications, they appear to be about the same as with cold-knife excision.

Again, you may experience some temporary localized pain, as well as some postsurgical bleeding. You'll have to take it easy for a few days or even a few weeks to allow the area to heal; your doctor may prescribe muscle relaxants or sitz baths to prevent anal sphincter spasm, a common side effect of the procedure. Always follow your doctor's postsurgical orders regarding resumption of regular physical and sexual activities, and be sure to return to your doctor for any follow-up screenings or checkups.

Anal Cancer

If anoscopic examination indicates that your disease has advanced beyond severe anal dysplasia—that the abnormal cells have begun to invade surrounding tissue—then the presence of invasive anal cancer is confirmed.

Anal cancer is very different from colon or rectal cancer, although they're often mixed up. Anal cancer occurs only in the anal epithelium, which includes the perianal region and the anal canal up to the *anorectal junction*, the area where the anus meets the rectum. Anal cancer is usually associated with HPV and therefore can be sexually acquired. In contrast, rectal and colon cancer are *not* associated with HPV and are *not* believed to be sexually acquired.

Colon and rectal cancer are much more common than anal cancer. In fact, if you're over the age of fifty, or if you have a family history of colon or rectum cancer and are over the age of forty, you should have a routine colonoscopy to rule out cancer or precancer in these areas. A colonoscopy is basically the insertion of a flexible scope up the anal canal, into the rectum, and all the way to the beginning part of the colon. It's done to visualize and biopsy areas that might be suspicious for cancer or precancer. However, a colonoscopy does not assess the anal area, and anal lesions are often missed. Conversely, remember that HRA only assesses the area up to the anorectal junction and does not assess colon or rectal cancer.

Symptoms of Anal Cancer

Any one or combination of the following symptoms can indicate invasive anal cancer: persistent swelling or itchiness in the anus, bleeding (even a small amount), pain or pressure in the area around the anus, discharge, or a lump near the anus. Talk to your doctor if you experience these symptoms, and he or she will call you in for an anal examination and anoscopy. Since some of these symptoms may also reflect a problem in the rectum or colon, if your doctor does not see any problems in the anus, you may also need a thorough evaluation of the colon and rectum.

Staging of Anal Cancer

Once invasive anal cancer is confirmed, your physician will begin the staging process. (Methods used in staging are covered on pages 151–156.) Staging allows your physician and oncologist to properly treat your cancer.

Stage	What It Means
0	Also known as carcinoma in situ (a variant of severe anal dysplasia), these cancerous cells are only found in the top layer of tissue. This is not really a form of anal cancer.
I	The cancer has spread beyond the top layer of anal tissue, is smaller than 2 cm in diameter, but has not spread to the muscle tissue of the anal sphincter.
II	Cancer has spread beyond the top layer of anal tissue, is larger than 2 cm in diameter, but has not spread to nearby organs or lymph nodes.
III-A	Cancer has spread to the lymph nodes around the rectum or to nearby organs such as the vagina or bladder.
III-B	Cancer has spread to the lymph nodes in the middle of the abdomen or in the groin, or the cancer has spread to both nearby organs and the lymph nodes around the rectum.
IV	Cancer has spread to distant lymph nodes within the abdomen or to organs in other parts of the body.
Recurrent	The cancer has come back in the anus or elsewhere after treatment.

Treatment

Treatment of anal cancer depends on the stage of the cancer and the patient's age and general health. (The special needs of HIV-positive patients will be covered in chapter 14.)

Stage 0

Also classified as anal carcinoma in situ, severe anal dysplasia, and AIN 3, the lesion will probably be removed using one of the treatments listed in the section on treatment of anal dysplasia.

Stage I

This fairly localized cancer can sometimes be treated by local resection, similar to Stage 0. However, the usual therapy is a combination of chemotherapy with radiation therapy. This therapy is quite effective and most of the time it does not lead to a colostomy (the surgical creation of a hole through which waste can pass). If cancer cells remain following therapy, abdominoperineal resection may remove the remaining cancer. In this procedure the entire anal canal is removed and a colostomy bag is required.

Stage II

The anal cancer is slightly larger but has not metastasized in Stage II. Treatment options are the same as for Stage I.

Stage III-A

Radiation plus chemotherapy is still an option, but because the cancer has spread to the lymph nodes, your physician may use surgery to remove parts of the rectum or colon as well as lymph node dissection followed by radiation therapy.

Stage III-B

In Stage III-B, the cancer has spread to both lymph nodes and nearby organs, so radiation and chemotherapy, followed by surgery, is the best combination. The type of surgery depends on how many cancer cells exist after the chemotherapy and radiation therapy, ranging from local resection to abdominoperineal resection. Lymph node dissection can be used to determine if the cancer has spread.

Stage IV

The cure rate of Stage IV anal cancer is low. The cancer has spread to distant organs and lymph nodes, and most treatments are palliative (designed to relieve symptoms rather than cure the cancer). Surgery, radiation, and chemotherapy all offer palliative benefits, and at this point, the patient should consider clinical trials or experimental therapies.

Recurrent

Recurrent anal cancer therapies usually depend on the original treatment: If cells came back after surgery, then radiation will probably be prescribed, and vice versa. In addition, patients with recurrent cancer should consider clinical trials.

Treatment Options for Anal Cancer

Radiation Therapy

Radiation therapy uses radiation to kill cancer cells. While normal cells are affected by radiation, they bounce back fairly soon; cancer cells are too weak to resist radiation. Side effects and methods of radiation therapy are covered in detail in chapter 7.

When the radiation beam is aimed at the anal canal and rectum, *radiation proctitis* can occur. This is severe inflammation of the anus and rectum and is sometimes associated with pain and bleeding with bowel movements. Usually this eases with time, but occasionally the side effects can be permanent. Sitz baths, anti-inflammatories, hydrocortisone enemas, zinc oxide cream, and stool softeners can offer some symptomatic relief.

Chemotherapy

Chemotherapy uses drugs to kill the cancer. Most of the time these are given intravenously. The drugs used most often for chemotherapy of anal cancer are 5-fluorouracil and mitomycin C. The main side effects of mitomycin C are damage to the bone marrow, loss of appetite, and decreased fertility. Other less common side effects include nausea and vomiting; damage to the liver, lungs, or kidneys; changes in the nails; mouth sores; diarrhea; and rarely alopecia (hair loss). Another drug that is increasingly being used is cisplatin. Detailed information on chemotherapy, including the possible side effects of 5-fluorouracil and cisplatin, is given on pp. 168–172.

Abdominoperineal Resection

Although abdominoperineal resection used to be the most common treatment for anal cancer, it's been used less and less as radiation and chemotherapy improve. This surgery removes the anus and lower part of the rectum by cutting into the abdomen and perineum. Afterwards, a surgeon will make an opening on the outside of the body through which waste can pass, called a colostomy. A colostomy bag is attached to the opening with a special type of glue and will collect the waste. Patients usually empty and take care of the colostomy bag themselves. Due to the extensive nature of this surgery—and its unpleasant aftereffects—abdominoperineal resection is usually done only if radiation and chemotherapy have not worked.

Lymph Node Dissection

Lymph node dissection simply involves the removal of lymph nodes to determine if the disease has spread and it may help to prevent the spread of cancer. It's usually done during or after abdominoperineal resection and is a fairly simple procedure.

Clinical Trials

Dozens of cancer centers conduct clinical trials, and they're often a good way for advanced or recurrent cancer patients to try new therapies. Your doctor can usually refer you to current clinical trials, and more details on clinical trials are covered in chapter 7.

Prevention of Anal Dysplasia and Anal Cancer

Assuming you're reading this because you already have HPV, you can't go back and prevent initial infection. But you *can* do some things to prevent reactivation of the virus and the development and progression of anal disease.

Improving your general health can both fight off current HPV infection and help prevent future lesions from forming. Lifestyle changes like quitting smoking, improving your nutrition, and exercising will boost your immunity, whether or not you're HIV-positive.

Condoms for anal intercourse may be used to prevent HPV transmission, not to mention most other sexually transmitted diseases, including HIV and HSV. Remember that while condoms do help, they're far from foolproof in preventing HPV transmission. However, they are a whole lot better than nothing, and they are effective at preventing transmission of HIV. Even if you already have HPV infection, preventing infection with new HPV types is probably important. Research studies often show more than one HPV type in the anal canal, especially among MSM, and this may indicate transmission from several partners.

Risk Factors

Like cervical cancer, the development of anal cancer or anal dysplasia is not solely dependent on HPV infection. Smoking remains a factor, and suppressed immunity is a major cause, especially among patients with HIV infection or those who are immunosuppressed by medication they are taking to prevent rejection of transplanted organs such as kidneys. Below is a list of risk factors for developing anal dysplasia. Remember that all of the risk factors for HPV also apply to anal dysplasia.

Risk Factors for Anal Dysplasia

- **HPV infection.** HPV infection is directly related to anal dysplasia.
- **High-risk sexual activities.** High-risk activities include unprotected receptive anal sex, but HPV can also be spread by fingers or inert objects, such as toys or dildos, that have come in contact with the virus.
- **Smoking.** Cigarette smoke contains carcinogens that both lower immunity and increase your chance of developing cancerous cells.
- **Lowered immunity due to HIV infection or other factors.** Although HIV is by far the most common immune disorder linked to anal dysplasia, other immunosuppressed conditions—such as pregnancy or recent organ transplant—can lead to anal dysplasia.
- **Poor general health.** Poor general nutrition and health lowers your body's natural defenses and may allow HPV to develop into anal dysplasia.
- **Poor health care.** Infrequent screenings and doctor visits could allow mild anal dysplasia to develop into severe anal dysplasia or cancer.

Conclusion

Like cervical cancer, anal cancer may be a preventable disease if it's caught in the anal dysplasia stage. Anal HPV infection and anal dysplasia are very common among high-risk women. If you belong to one of the high-risk groups discussed earlier in this chapter, talk to your doctor about being screened and treated. In the meantime, if you continue engaging in high-risk sexual activities, use protection. Condoms can help prevent HPV infection, not to mention other infections such as HIV.

Talking to Your Doctor about Anal Dysplasia

This might be extraordinarily difficult for a number of reasons. Trying to tell your doctor that you belong to one of the high-risk groups may be embarrassing, and you may fear being judged. Talking about anal sexual activity triggers all kinds of emotions. Another big issue is that, having read this book, I suspect that you now know more about anal dysplasia than your doctor—you might have do some educating here.

Below is a list of questions that you should ask your doctor:

Questions to Ask Your Doctor

- Do you know how to do an anal Pap smear? If not, can you refer me to someone who does?

- Do you know how to do high resolution anoscopy? If not, can you refer me to someone who does?
- What did my anal Pap smear and/or anal biopsy show?
- What kind of treatment procedure will I have? What is the advantage of this treatment over the other available treatments?
- What if I choose not to be treated for my anal dysplasia, but to be followed? What are the risks?
- What is the success rate of your recommended treatment?
- If I need to be referred to a surgeon for treatment, does he or she know how to do high resolution anoscopy? Is he or she experienced in the treatment of anal dysplasia?
- Should I bring a friend with me for my treatment?
- Will I experience any side effects?
- Was all of the abnormal tissue removed?
- What should I do to lessen the side effects of my procedure?
- When should I come for my follow-up Pap smear?
- How often after my initial follow-up should I come in?
- What can I do to prevent anal dysplasia?
- What should I tell my partner?
- Does my partner need to be examined?

PART FOUR

Benign HPV Infection

CHAPTER ELEVEN

Genital Warts

Thus far, I've devoted most of this book to oncogenic HPV types and the diseases they can cause. Oncogenic HPV infections are particularly insidious, since they're often subclinical and escape recognition until cancer has developed. On the other hand, the consequences of oncogenic HPV infection can often be controlled if it's caught early on—for instance, if you have severe dysplasia, removal with LEEP or simple laser surgery can possibly prevent cervical cancer. Although you still may carry the virus, and it could reactivate under certain circumstances, recurrence is rare, and with vigilance, development of serious disease in the future is rare.

Now let's talk about nononcogenic HPV types. These are often called the "benign" or "low-risk" HPV types. Nononcogenic HPVs have their good side: Namely, they don't cause cancer. The most common genital HPV types linked with warts, 6 and 11, rarely cause lethal conditions (except respiratory papillomatosis, covered in the next chapter). However, nononcogenic HPV causes the frequently recurrent *condyloma acuminata*, also known as genital warts. Oncogenic HPV types such as 16 or 18 *do* occasionally cause genital warts.

Other common benign HPV types are types 1, 2, and 4. These are the HPV types that cause warts in the skin of the hands and feet. As you recall, HPV 6 and 11 rarely, if ever, stray outside the genital region, and HPV types 1, 2, and 4 only rarely show up in the genital epithelium. If you have a wart on your hands or feet, and you or your partner have warts in the genital region, chances are that these lesions aren't related.

Why learn about genital warts if they don't cause cancer and they don't kill you? Although genital warts aren't fatal, they cause a lot of misery. They can burn, itch, or bleed. They look unsightly and they're embarrassing. They also cost a lot of money—our health care system pays hundreds of millions of dollars each year to get rid of them.

Genital Warts 101

Most of what you need to know about how HPV works is included in chapter 1, "HPV 101." The trauma of sexual intercourse can cause small tears and abrasions in the mucous membranes, and this might permit HPV to enter the basal cell layer. In many cases, HPV will never do more than infect a few cells and remain latent; many young people never exhibit lesions due to HPV, and if they do, they go away on their own. The reason why some people develop warts and some don't is not known, but cigarette smoking and compromised immunity almost certainly play roles for some people. Then again, the healthiest person in the world might still develop genital warts.

The development of warts usually begins within three months after transmission and can develop on any region of contact; the cervix, vagina, vulva, penis, and anus are the most common starting points for wart growth.

As a reminder, warts are lesions that are usually bumpy and that, when examined under the microscope, show special cells called *koilocytes*. Not all warts are bumpy, though; some are flat. From a classification point of view, warts belong to the category of low-grade disease, like mild cervical or anal dysplasia. Warts are often covered by *keratin*, a thick layer of protein produced by the epithelial cells. Warts that have a lot of it are called *hyperkeratotic,* and this presents a problem because the thick keratin layer sometimes prevents penetration of topical treatments for the warts, rendering them ineffective. Apart from the symptoms of the warts, their clinical significance is twofold: (1) They signify an increased risk of having other HPV types, including oncogenic HPV types, in other parts of the anogenital tract, and (2) warts contain the largest numbers of mature HPV particles, and this is the stage at which HPV is most easily transmitted to a sexual partner.

Cervical Genital Warts

Cervical warts are probably less common than warts on the outer genital regions. Unlike warts on the external genitals such as the vulva and even the vagina, which usually contain HPV 6 or 11, warts on the cervix may also contain HPV types 42, 43, and 44. Cervical warts can only be diagnosed by your doctor; a Pap smear will likely show LSIL, and when your doctor performs a colposcopy (outlined on pages 98–101), he or she will probably see exophytic (out from the surface) warts in your cervix. She may also see flat warts. As is the case with mild, moderate, and severe dysplasia, the application of acetic acid will turn warts white, making them more visible to the naked eye. Your doctor may be able to see cervical genital warts during a regular pelvic examination if they have grown exophytically.

Although genital warts do *not* cause cervical cancer, the existence of warts growing in your cervix indicates active HPV infection and indicates that you may be contagious. So you may want to discuss immediate treatment with your doctor. Often, cervical warts, like mild dysplasia in general, regress to normal in a few months on their own. Once they're gone, you're less likely to be infectious, even if you continue to have HPV infection. And remember, if you have cervical warts with one of the low-risk HPV types, you may be at risk of having some of the oncogenic HPV types as well.

Symptoms of Cervical Warts

Although you won't experience any physical symptoms of cervical warts, your doctor will be able to recognize them by sight during a colposcopy. They may be single or multiple; scattered or lumped together in one area. They're usually found within your transformation zone, but may also grow on your outer cervix. They can also grow and spread into the endocervical canal, which leads up to the uterus. If, during a colposcopy, your doctor can't see the entire lesion—that is, it may have spread into the endocervical canal—he or she may perform an endocervical curettage, described on page 101.

Treatment of Cervical Warts

The initial phase of your workup will be aimed at determining if you have any lesions more advanced than warts, since that may change the therapy. If nothing other than cervical warts is found, the treatment options include LEEP, laser surgery, and cryotherapy (described in chapter 6). TCA and Efudex may be used as well. Aggressive surgery, including conization, should be used only if the genital warts are excessive or recurrent. The less surgery that's done on your cervix, the better, which is why many doctors recommend waiting to see if your body's natural defenses can fight off the warts. As with any HPV-associated lesion, pregnancy and immunosuppression can increase the number and size of the warts, and this may complicate the therapy. In many instances you may choose to defer therapy until after the pregnancy is completed and the immune system has had a chance to return to normal.

Vaginal Warts

Vaginal HPV infection is often linked to vulvar or cervical HPV. Often the infection may originate on the vulva or within the cervix and spread into the vagina. If you have vulvar or cervical condylomas, you should have a careful vaginal examination as well. Because a speculum often covers lesions during a regular pelvic exam, your physician should carefully examine the walls of the vagina while removing the speculum. Colposcopy can also identify smaller lesions. As with cervical warts, vaginal warts may become more problematic with pregnancy.

Symptoms of Vaginal Warts

Vaginal warts are usually asymptomatic, although a woman may also experience vaginal discharge and severe, persistent itching (*pruritis* in medicalese). Occasionally, patients may bleed after sex.

Condylomas are often multiple in the vagina, with patchy distribution; the upper and lower thirds are most commonly affected, possibly in relation to vulvar or cervical infection (Campion et al. 1996). If you regularly self-examine your vagina, you may notice the lesions themselves, which are rough, dense, white elevations, although most vaginal infections aren't plainly visible to the naked eye. (See appendix B on vaginal self-exams.) Even when they are, they could be mistaken for the normal ridges and bumps of your vaginal wall. In any case, application of vinegar may lead to acetowhitening of the lesions, which may then be easily identified during colposcopy.

Treatment of Vaginal Warts

Again, many doctors opt for the wait-and-see method of treatment. On the other hand, many women want their warts treated as soon as possible. Sometimes when lesions are treated in the cervix or vulva, vaginal lesions go away as well. Therapies for vaginal warts include cryosurgery, laser vaporization, and topical medication. Detailed information on treatment is covered in the next chapter.

Vulvar Warts

Vulvar condylomas are the most familiar, most tenacious expression of genital warts in women. In the last fifteen years, the United States has experienced a 150 percent increase of vulvar wart cases, and that increase is especially evident in women between the ages of sixteen and twenty-five years. Unlike cervical HPV, most cases of vulvar HPV lead to the formation of condylomata acuminata, or genital warts. A photo of vulvar warts is shown in figure 11.1.

Symptoms of Vulvar Warts

The vulva is a large area, including the labia majora and minora, clitoris, vestibule, mons, and vaginal opening, and each area consists of a different type of surface.

The vestibule, vagina, and cervix are lined by mucous membranes. Warts in these areas tend to be fleshy and vascular in appearance, and are best recognized through acetowhitening.

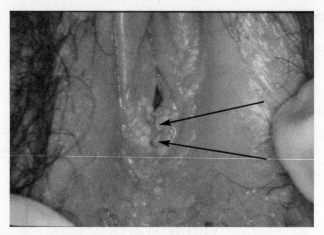

Figure 11.1: Vulvar Warts. *This photo shows multiple small warts (condyloma acuminatum) on the vulva (see arrows). (Photo courtesy of Dr. Anna-Barbara Moscicki, University of California, San Francisco.)*

The labia minora, clitoris, and interlabial area are covered by lightly keratinized, slightly tougher skin. Warts here are soft, white, and bumpy and can often be seen with the naked eye or felt with your finger.

The labia majora (the two larger lips protecting the inner vulva) and mons pubis (the surrounding pubic area) are covered by keratinized skin. This skin grows coarse, curly pubic hair, and has roughly the same consistency as other areas of the body. Warts here are keratotic—meaning they are harder and rougher—and they're often skin-colored.

Vulvar warts most commonly occur in the moist areas, including the labia minora and vaginal opening. Mucous membranes are especially vulnerable, since they provide so much opportunity for infection; cells shed and create an ideal environment for genital warts. You'll probably notice the changes to your vulva before your doctor does, and if not, he or she will certainly recognize them during a pelvic exam. Warts in the vulvar area are associated with the same symptoms as warts elsewhere—burning, itching, and bleeding. Of course, they may also be totally asymptomatic.

Treatment of Vulvar Warts

Because vulvar warts are on the outside of your body (with the exception of infection that has spread to the lower vagina), topical medications are usually the best first line of defense. Detailed information on these and other treatments is given in the next chapter.

Recurrence

Recurrent infection is common, no matter how successful the treatment is. Therapies only treat the warts, not HPV itself. Vulvar warts can be extremely tenacious, and recurrence rates reach up to 50 percent. Your body's immunity affects the growth of warts, and if you're pregnant, HIV-positive, or suffer another immune disorder, warts tend to grow much faster and larger (Boxman et al. 1999). One study has shown that HPV DNA has even been found in pubic hair, but keep in mind that shaving pubic hair is one method of transmission—frequent nicks or abrasions could lead to more warts.

HPV, oncogenic or benign, can be latent for long periods of time before reactivating. We may see high recurrence rates with genital warts simply because they're visible; cervical infection can also come and go, but you just don't see it happening.

Perianal Warts and Warts in the Anal Canal

In about 18 percent of patients with vulvar or penile warts, infection can spread to the perineum, perianal area, or anal canal. Touching or scratching warts in one part of your genital region, followed by touching or scratching another area, such as the anal region, could spread the infection to that area. In addition, the usual culprits, such as anal intercourse, fingers, toys, etc., can also lead to infection of the anal area with HPV. It's also possible that intra-anal disease (disease in the anal canal) may occur even in the absence of any kind of anal penetration, since HPV introduced into the perianal tissues (outside the anal canal, surrounding the opening of the anus) could conceivably migrate upward on its own. As with vulvar warts, these can be spread by shaving.

Most perianal warts are associated with HPV 6 or 11, but warts inside the anal canal are associated with a wider variety of HPV types.

Regarding treatment of anal warts, it's most helpful to think separately about perianal and intra-anal warts. Warts in the perianal region are treated in much the same way as those of the vulva (topically or surgically), but they're often larger and can create other symptoms such as bleeding. They can also itch or burn. As with vaginal or vulvar warts indicating increased likelihood of cervical disease, anal warts are a harbinger of other lesions inside the anal canal. You may therefore want to discuss HRA with your doctor to rule out intra-anal dysplasia.

Treatment of perianal warts is similar to that of vulvar warts and usually begins with topical medications. Detailed information on these and other treatments is given in the next chapter. Treatment of intra-anal warts is more challenging because of the internal location. Essentially these are treated the same way as anal dysplasia.

Risk Factors for Genital Warts

The risk factors for acquiring HPV are listed in chapter 1, but development of genital warts include a few more factors that bear listing here.

Risk Factors for Developing Genital Warts

- **HPV 6 or 11 infection.** Oncogenic HPV types can cause genital warts, but not as often as HPV 6 or 11. Of course, the risk of infection increases with exposure to a partner with warts. Uncircumcised men often show a higher prevalence of genital warts than circumcised men.
- **Poor hygiene.** Warts thrive in warm, moist surfaces. Good hygiene, including keeping the skin dry, will help to prevent the growth of warts.
- **Low immunity.** Pregnancy, HIV infection, and organ transplant treatments often lead to lower immunity; patients with these conditions often exhibit persistent, confluent genital warts.
- **The presence of other STDs.** Other STDs may weaken local immunity and may increase HPV replication.
- **Poor health care.** Warts that are left untreated may go away on their own, but they may also spread the virus and cause a more severe infection. Suspicious lesions should be examined by a doctor.
- **Smoking.** Smoking cigarettes decreases both general and local immunity to HPV.

Conclusion

With proper treatment, improved general health, and safer sexual practices, warts usually go away at least temporarily, with recurrence in about half the cases. Eventually, with repeated attempts at therapy, most patients are successful in ridding themselves of warts. In the meantime, remember that warts represent a highly infectious form of HPV infection. You might consider abstaining from sexual activity or using condoms while you continue to have untreated or incompletely treated warts.

While rarely life-threatening, developing genital warts can be a traumatic, unpleasant experience. Many patients find great comfort in talking with other HPV sufferers, so ask your physician about support groups, either online or in your neighborhood. Chapter 15 of this book, "Living with HPV and Talking with Your Partner," covers many of the emotional issues you may experience.

Questions to Ask Your Doctor

- Where are my warts?
- Was my cervical Pap smear normal?
- Should I have an anal Pap smear?
- What is the best treatment method for my warts?
- How long will the treatment last?
- What is the success rate of the treatment?
- What are the side effects of the treatment?
- How much will the treatment cost?

- How long will I need to be followed to make sure the warts are really gone?
- What should I tell my partner?
- Should my partner be examined?
- What can I do to prevent future warts?

CHAPTER TWELVE

Methods of Treatment for Genital Warts

The treatment of genital warts usually depends on the severity and persistence of the symptoms, the chances of recurrence, and your own desires as a patient. If only one wart exists, then you and your physician might decide to wait on treatment. Many genital warts regress on their own and never come back. If one or two warts persist, but remain unchanged, you may or may not decide to treat them at that point, depending on your sexual activity. If the warts increase in size and number, though, you'll probably want to seek treatment sooner rather than later.

In addition, if *any* vulvar warts are visible, your doctor should carefully examine your vagina, cervix, perineum, and anus for evidence of further infection (18 percent of patients with vulvar warts also have warts on the perineum and anus). Likewise, if your partner has warts on his penis, the scrotum, pubic area, perineum, and anus should also be examined.

If your warts do not respond to treatment, your doctor may want to biopsy them to rule out more advanced disease like severe vulvar or vaginal dysplasia, or verrucous carcinoma, a form of squamous cell cancer that has some warty features.

Treatment for genital warts falls into two categories: patient-applied and provider (doctor)-administered. Patient-applied treatments include topical creams (podofilox and imiquimod) that you can get a prescription for, take home, and apply yourself. Provider-administered therapies involve more delicate, skilled procedures, including cryosurgery, podophyllin resin, trichloroacetic acid (TCA), bichloroacetic acid, interferon, and surgery.

Deciding which treatment to use depends on wart size, number, and location, as well as your preference, the cost of the treatment, convenience, any special circumstances (such as pregnancy or HIV infection), and your doctor's personal preference. For instance, warts on the moist areas respond well to topical treatment, while drier warts tend to need a different approach, including cryotherapy. In addition, if you're pregnant, most patient-applied therapies are not recommended.

Most genital wart patients require more than one treatment application, so you and your doctor need to come up with the best plan for completely eradicating the warts. Most outbreaks require multiple provider-administered treatments or self-administered treatments, and many plans of therapy combine both.

Table 12.1 shows the most common therapies for the various types of genital warts.

Rates of efficacy and recurrence are quoted from the STD Treatment Guidelines from the U.S. Centers for Disease Control and Prevention.

Patient-Applied Therapies

Patient-applied therapies usually come in a solution, gel, or cream and can be applied at home. They're the least expensive, most convenient treatment and are usually considered to be the first line of defense. If you don't respond to a patient-applied therapy within the allotted time (usually from four to eight weeks, depending on the drug), your doctor may opt for a provider-administered treatment.

Keep in mind, though, that up to 50 percent of patients may experience recurrence of warts about six months after treatment. Recurrence doesn't mean that your treatment was unsuccessful; it only means that the virus still exists in your skin and has reactivated. Also, if some of your warts were too small to see, or difficult to apply the cream to, you may not have treated them in the first place. During recurrence, you may use the same or a different therapy as before.

Note: Patient-applied therapies are *not* recommended for pregnant women, and women at risk of becoming pregnant must use at least one effective method of birth control while being treated.

Table 12.1.

THERAPIES FOR GENITAL WARTS

	Podofilox*	Imiquimod*	Podophyllin*	TCA	Cryotherapy	Electrosurgery**	Surgical Excision	Laser Surgery	LEEP	5-FU*	Notes
Vulvar/Perianal	X	X	X	X	X	X	X	X	X		
Cervical					X	X		X	X	X	dysplasia must be ruled out before therapy commences
Vaginal			X	X	X					X	
Urethral Meatus			X	X	X					X	
Intra-anal				X	X	X	X	X			
Oral					X	X	X				

* Contraindicated for pregnant women

** Contraindicated for patients with pacemakers

Podofilox 0.5 Percent Solution or Gel

Podofilox, a drug that prevents cells from dividing, destroys warts and is inexpensive, simple to use, and safe. Its trade name is Condylox. Podofilox is the purified active ingredient (podophyllotoxin) in a solution called podophyllin resin, which was used quite commonly in the past for treatment of warts (see page 274). About 88 percent of patients respond to podofilox, but recurrence can occur in up to 60 percent of cases.

Your doctor will show you the best way to apply the medication before you take it home yourself, and he or she will also indicate which warts should be treated. Since podofilox should not be applied to an area greater than 10 square centimeters, and since many warts go away on their own, your doctor will probably tell you to treat only the largest, most persistent warts. In addition, keratinized warts on dry areas may not respond as well to podofilox as warts in moister areas.

Solutions require a cotton swab, while the gel can be applied with your finger. The warts should be completely visible for application, so you might want to use a mirror and light for guidance.

Podofilox requires application twice a day for three days, then four days with no therapy. If the warts do not go away or decrease in size or number after the first treatment, the cycle of three days on, four days off, can be repeated up to four times. You may experience mild to moderate pain or local irritation after treatment. If the warts remain after a month of treatment, you and your physician may choose another therapy route.

Again, podofilox is not safe to use during pregnancy.

Imiquimod 5 Percent Cream

Imiquimod is another inexpensive, simple topical treatment and recently has shown evidence of being even more effective than podofilox. Its trade name is Aldara. It acts as an immune enhancer that is believed to work by stimulating local production of interferon to fight the virus. Inteferons are naturally occurring proteins secreted in response to virus infections. Since it became available in the late 1990s, imiquimod has shown encouraging results and may even be useful in patients who did not respond well to podofilox.

Imiquimod can be applied by finger at bedtime, three times a week, for up to sixteen weeks. The treated area should be washed off with mild soap and water about six to ten hours after application to prevent excessive irritation.

About 50 percent of imiquimod users are clear of warts by eight to ten weeks or sooner, and about 75 percent show partial clearance of warts. In addition, the recurrence rate is lower than for other topical treatments (Perry and Lamb 1999).

Provider (Doctor)-Administered Therapies

If topical treatments are unsuccessful, if warts recur frequently, or if you're pregnant, you and your doctor may opt for a provider-administered therapy. Provider-administered therapies are also better options than patient-applied therapies if the warts are too small or difficult to reach for the patient. These therapies require a visit to your doctor's office and are more expensive and inconvenient than topical treatment. They are, however, effective in treating warts and are a good alternative to patient-applied therapies.

Cryotherapy

Cryotherapy uses liquid nitrogen or a cryoprobe to freeze off warts. As far as surgical procedures go, it's relatively inexpensive and doesn't require anesthesia, although you may experience moderate pain during and after the procedure. If performed properly, it shouldn't cause any scarring, either, which can occur with some other procedures. In addition, cryotherapy is a safe treatment for pregnant women.

The cryotherapy should be reapplied every one or two weeks, depending on how quickly you heal from the previous treatment. It's most effective on keratinized warts, the rougher, harder warts on the dry, hairy areas of your genitals, although it can also be used for the moister areas. Up to 88 percent of cryotherapy patients have successful treatment, with about 40 percent of patients experiencing a recurrence.

Trichloroacetic Acid (TCA)

TCA, an 80 percent to 90 percent acidic solution, is similar in efficacy to cryotherapy and also is not contraindicated during pregnancy. It is similar to another acid used by some doctors, known as bichloroacetic acid. Your doctor will apply a small amount of TCA to warts and allow it to dry, causing a white frosting-like substance to develop on the wart. You may experience mild to moderate pain during therapy, but most patients experience a feeling of heat. The discomfort is usually minor and fades in less than thirty minutes, and an application of baking soda may be used to remove unreacted acid. Care must be taken to minimize exposure of normal epithelium to TCA. TCA may also lead to more scarring than liquid nitrogen.

If necessary, your physician may repeat the treatment once a week for up to six applications; if warts persist after six weeks, you should seek other therapies. The success rate of TCA is about 80 percent, with recurrences among 36 percent of patients. TCA can be administered with caution to pregnant women.

Electrodessication and Electrocautery

Electrodessication and electrocautery use an electric current to destroy or remove warts. Because of their expense and the equipment required—you'll need local anesthesia, as well as a skilled doctor—they're considered a second-line therapy. Patients rarely try electrodessication unless a previous therapy has failed.

The primary benefit of electrosurgery is that the warts are removed immediately and repeat visits may not be necessary. In addition, bleeding and scarring are minimal. Recurrence occurs in 22 percent of patients, and electrosurgery is contraindicated for patients with cardiac pacemakers or lesions near the opening of the anus to the outside.

Podophyllin Resin

Podophyllin resin is a smelly, somewhat unstable solution whose active ingredient is podophyllotoxin, the main component of Condylox, described above. It's applied to the warts and, like podofilox, is toxic. Like cryotherapy and TCA, it's relatively inexpensive, simple, and safe, but may require more therapy sessions than other treatments. Podophyllin may cause mild to moderate pain or local irritation after treatment, and it can be toxic; you'll need to thoroughly wash the area one to four hours after treatment. The application should therefore be applied to the lesions *only,* with an effort to limit exposure of the normal skin. If necessary, you'll have to return for therapy once a week, and if warts persist after six applications, you and your doctor should discuss alternative therapy. Heavily keratinized warts may not respond as well as mucosal warts. The success rate of podophyllin therapy can range from 32 percent to 79 percent, and about 27 percent to 65 percent of patients experience recurrences. With the advent of podofilox and imiquimod, and the availability of other, less toxic, provider-applied medications such as TCA or liquid nitrogen, the use of podophyllin has declined somewhat in the last few years.

Note: Podophyllin should *not* be administered to pregnant women, and women at risk of becoming pregnant must use at least one effective method of birth control while being treated.

Surgical Excision

Like electrosurgery, surgical excision is considered a second-line therapy because it requires a skilled doctor, local anesthetic, and a longer office visit than topical therapies. The trade-off is that it usually renders you wart-free in one visit, and it's most beneficial for patients with a larger number or area of genital warts.

Warts can be removed with tangential excision with a pair of fine scissors or a scalpel, or by curettage. The resulting wound extends only into the top layer of skin. If the surgery is done properly, you won't need any sutures, and healing takes about the same amount of time as any other type of cut into the skin. Recurrences depend on the patient's immunity, and occur in about 29 percent of cases. Surgical excision is safe for most patients.

Carbon Dioxide Lasers

Carbon dioxide lasers are an alternative to surgical excision or electrosurgery for extensive warts and warts inside the urethra, particularly for patients who haven't responded to other treatments. Again, it's expensive and requires a skilled doctor but removes the warts in one visit and heals quickly. Recurrence does occur frequently, so discuss alternatives with your doctor. Lasers are safe for most patients.

Interferon Therapy

You may read about interferons in your treatment research. They stimulate local immunity to allow your body to kill warts (Imiquimod, a topical therapy I mentioned earlier, stimulates your body's interferons [Reid 1996]).

With interferon therapy, the doctor injects interferon either directly into the base of a wart, and the success and recurrence rates are comparable to other therapies. However, most doctors don't recommend interferon therapy, since it's expensive, inconvenient, requires many office visits, and is associated with a high rate of recurrence and adverse effects. Any benefits from interferon therapy can usually be obtained through more convenient, safer, less expensive routes.

5-Fluorouracil Cream

More widely known for its use in cancer chemotherapy, 5-fluorouracil, when put into topical cream form, has been used to treat vaginal and sometimes vulvar warts. Its trade name is Efudex, and I have already discussed its use in the treatment of vaginal and vulvar dysplasia (see chapters 8 and 9). Applied with a vaginal applicator, 5-fluorouracil cream can be quite effective when it's used properly.

Use of 5-fluorouracil cream has declined somewhat in the last few years with the advent of other, less toxic treatments. Application of just a little too much can lead to ulceration of the epithelium. So while it works pretty well, the incidence of side effects is also high. For this reason, 5-fluorouracil cream is also considered by many doctors to be second-line therapy.

Note: 5-fluorouracil cream should *not* be administered to pregnant women, and women at risk of becoming pregnant must use at least one effective method of birth control while being treated.

Follow-up Treatments

Even if you're using a patient-applied therapy, you should visit your doctor several times during treatment. You'll want to monitor the disappearance of warts as well as treat any complications of therapy, and education and counseling are important aspects of therapy. High stress levels can lessen your immunity and encourage wart growth.

After you're clear of all visible genital warts, you should watch for recurrences; they usually occur during the first three months after therapy, but can occur any time thereafter. Overall, the risk of recurrence declines somewhat after the first year, so I recommend a follow-up evaluation three months after treatment, and at least once more within the following nine months.

Conclusion

Although all of these treatments present a range of benefits and drawbacks, none of them guarantee that you'll be rid of genital warts forever. The good news is that with enough persistence, eventually most patients are successful in getting rid of the warts. Recurrences frequently occur, but the nature of HPV prevents us from knowing if it's a true recurrence, caused by the previous infection, reinfection with the same HPV type, or even infection with a new one.

Practicing safe sex can reduce, but not eliminate, the risk of reinfection and transmission to uninfected partners. In addition, keep in mind that although genital warts aren't usually caused by high-risk HPV types, they could indicate the presence of other HPV types elsewhere in the anogenital epithelium. Regular cervical Pap smears should be performed to rule out cervical warts and dysplasia.

CHAPTER THIRTEEN

Recurrent Respiratory Papillomatosis

An unusual but potentially life-threatening complication of genital HPV infection is a disease known as *recurrent respiratory papillomatosis*, or RRP. This disease can occur when HPV is transmitted at birth. As I mentioned earlier, the hormonal imbalances and loss of immunity during pregnancy often cause florid HPV expression—that is, a woman who may occasionally experience one or two genital warts may suddenly develop widespread warts throughout her vulva, vagina, and even cervix. The danger of pregnancy-associated genital warts is twofold. First, large genital warts in the vagina and vulva could obstruct the birth canal or cause excessive bleeding during delivery. Fortunately this is exceedingly rare. Second, HPV can be passed along to the newborn during birth. Although we're not sure exactly when transmission occurs, studies indicate that the chance of transmission increases with increased time between your water breaking and delivery. (Tenti et al. 1999) This is far more likely to happen when you have active HPV infection in the form of genital warts than if you are shedding HPV in the absence of any detectable genital disease.

You might wonder if women who are known to have genital warts at the time of delivery should have a cesarean section to prevent transmission to the baby. Most experts agree that this usually isn't necessary. Although some cases of RRP could theoretically be prevented, the low frequency of RRP does not appear to justify use of this operation routinely, in view of the complications associated with cesarean section.

It's also possible that a woman with either active or inactive HPV infection is spreading HPV to her baby even if the baby shows no signs of RRP. In fact, several studies show that this happens quite often. However, it appears to cause few, if any, problems. Although HPVs can be found on the skin of newborns for several days after birth, in almost all cases, it becomes undetectable thereafter. The babies show no signs of disease and, in fact, show no evidence that they were ever truly infected. More likely the virus was just hanging out for a while on the surface of their skin for a few days without ever truly entering the cells. In medicalese we call that a *colonization.*

Overall, then, RRP appears to be a rare complication of a mom's infection with HPV 6 or 11 at the time of delivery. If it does occur, it can be devastating, and even potentially fatal. The open mouth of a newborn presents an ideal mucous membrane for HPV infection, and when the virus enters the mouth and throat, it can produce benign epithelial growths—warts—on the larynx and in the lungs.

Two types of RRP exist: juvenile-onset and adult-onset. The juvenile-onset form is more common and occurs in infants and young children, while the adult-onset form affects patients age eighteen and older. Although some cases of RRP are controlled after several surgical excisions, even small papillomas can block the narrow larynx of young children or even spread into the trachea (the windpipe) and the lungs. Some children require dozens of surgical procedures and never quite succeed in getting rid of the disease altogether. Others do fine, and as they grow older, their larynx and trachea enlarge in size, and perhaps they develop stronger immunity to HPV.

Transmission

As I said, we don't know exactly when vertical transmission—transmission from mother to newborn—occurs. Children born through vaginal *and* cesarean births have developed RRP, although the incidence is higher among vaginal births. HPV may enter through amniotic fluid after the water breaks, or when the newborn passes through the birth canal; we just don't know. If a woman has been recently diagnosed with condyloma, if she has an active infection, or if this is her first child, she may present a higher risk of transmission. There is no evidence to suggest that a mother can pass HPV to her unborn baby while the baby is still in the womb.

The risk of papillomatosis developing in children whose

mothers have HPV 6 or 11 is clearly higher than in the general population, but exactly how much higher is not known. Fortunately, the virus often clears in the first months after birth.

Unfortunately, we don't know yet why some infants clear infection and some develop RRP, or who is affected by juvenile-onset as opposed to adult-onset RRP. Some cases of adult-onset RRP may be related to intimate sexual contact, such as oral sex.

Juvenile-Onset RRP

Because warts grow on the larynx, hoarseness is the first, most common symptom. The growths are rarely painful, but older children may remark on the feeling that something's stuck in their throat, or that they're having difficulty breathing.

About 25 percent of patients are diagnosed in the first twelve months, and 50 percent to 75 percent are diagnosed before age 5. The other 25 percent develop between age five and adolescence.

If the infection goes unchecked, the warts can eventually block the airway; small children are at the highest risk for obstructed airways simply because their throats are smaller. In addition, papilloma infection can cause inflammatory swelling of the larynx and throat, which further blocks the air passage.

Because opening the passage with a tracheotomy can increase the risk of new lesions in the trachea, the only practical therapy for RRP is meticulous, painstaking surgical removal of the lesions. Often, the lesions can develop so quickly that surgery is required up to once a week.

In most cases, the need for frequent operations diminishes with age, and *recurrent* respiratory papilloma often ceases at or around puberty. Complete remission, though, is rare, and patients may experience regrowth from time to time.

Adult-Onset RRP

Adolescents rarely experience a new case of RRP. Around the age of twenty years, though, adult-onset RRP may develop. Again, hoarseness is the first symptom, and a patient may feel a lump in his or her throat. Adult-onset RRP is rarely as life-threatening as juvenile-onset. The growths are usually smaller and less frequent, so repeated surgeries are less necessary. One danger of adult-onset RRP is the potential for squamous cell carcinoma. Although HPV 6 and 11 are low-risk types, malignant transformation does very occasionally happen. In the past, some individuals with RRP were treated with radiation therapy to slow the growth of the lesions, and it's possible this may have increased the risk of progression to malignancy. In addition, cigarette smoking increases the risk for progression to cancer (Kashima, Mounts, and Shah 1996). Note, however, that the vast majority of squamous cell lung cancers have nothing to do with HPV infection.

Treatment

Treatment of RRP is primarily designed to alleviate the symptoms of the disease and to make the patient as comfortable as possible. With microlaryngoscopy, a procedure that shows the inside of a patient's throat, a surgeon uses a carbon dioxide laser to remove as much of the papilloma as possible without damaging the surrounding tissue.

Because surgery alone may leave subclinical or latent infection, many patients opt for combination therapy: surgical removal of warts in addition to antiviral and growth-inhibiting drugs such as interferons and retinoids. Although interferons are not effective in removing genital warts, long-term interferon therapy has achieved complete remission in 40 percent of cases and partial remission in an additional 40 percent (Kashima, Mounts, and Shah 1996).

Other forms of therapy also appear to be promising: Good results have been achieved in some patients with a drug called cidofovir and with a drug called indole-3 carbinol—one of the antioxidant substances in broccoli. As usual, your mother was right—you should eat your broccoli!

Risk Factors for RRP

- **HPV 6 or 11 infection in the mother.** Mother-to-child HPV transmission is necessary for RRP to develop. Young mothers with genital warts at the time of delivery of their first child are at the highest risk. Although latent infections occasionally pass on to newborns, women with active vaginal or vulvar infections are more at risk.
- **Longer time elapsed between water breaking and delivery.** Recent studies have shown that the longer the time elapsed

between initial water breaking and delivery, the more likely the newborn will be born with HPV.

- **Vaginal birth.** Although cesarean section doesn't rule out the possibility of transmission, vaginal birth—especially if the mother has an active infection—greatly increases the risk.
- **First-born infants.** First-born infants delivered to young women with HPV are most commonly afflicted with RRP.
- **Compromised immunity.** Immune disorders, such as HIV, can contribute to the development of RRP.
- **Intimate sexual contact.** Adult-onset RRP may be related to oral sex.

Risk Factors for Cancerous Changes in RRP

- **Smoking.** Cigarette smoking both influences the growth of warts in adult-onset RRP and contributes to laryngeal or lung cancer.
- **Radiation therapy.** Using irradiation to treat RRP increases the risk of malignant transformation.

Conclusion

Recurrent respiratory papillomatosis is a rare, but potentially fatal, condition. In addition to airway blockage, RRP causes great upheaval in the lives of parents and children. The surgery, expense, and general fear can be traumatic for the entire family. Talk to your doctor about joining a support group, or think about seeing a family or child counselor. One such group is called the Recurrent Respiratory Papillomatosis Foundation, and their Web site is *www.rrpf.org*. Juvenile-onset RRP usually fades by puberty, and adult-onset RRP poses a real danger only if the patient presents a high risk for cancer.

PART FIVE

Anal and Penile HPV Infections in Men

CHAPTER FOURTEEN

Men and HPV

Why have I included a chapter on HPV infection in men? With Pap smears in the title, I'd imagine a guy isn't likely to browse through this book. But since HPV is a sexually transmitted agent, and HPV causes lesions on the penis, I think it's important for women to understand the other half of the equation. I'm also *hoping* that men will read this book, and that they will get something out of it, too, either because they have signs or symptoms of HPV infection themselves, or they want to better understand what is going on with their partner.

This subject is challenging, to say the least. Compared to what we know about cervical HPV infection, we don't know much about HPV infection of the penis. In part, this is because it's much harder to study on the penis. The skin of the penis is keratinized, and among the various female genital organs, it probably resembles the skin of the vulva the most. Since it's not mucosal, it's too dry to allow for the penile equivalent of a Pap smear. Collecting a sample for HPV testing is similarly difficult.

In addition, while HPV contributes to the development of penile cancer, penile cancer is much less common than cervical cancer. A massive effort to identify potentially precancerous penile lesions has never been made because the lesions don't usually progress to cancer.

All in all, collecting detailed information on penile HPV infection has been much tougher than it has been for the cervix. That's a pity, since having this kind of information could be really helpful to controlling the HPV epidemic. As with any other epidemic of sexually transmitted agents, it makes sense to think about both the male and the female roles in transmission.

So what *do* we know? We know HPV can infect virtually anywhere on the skin of the penis, but the location varies according to whether or not the man is circumcised. Uncircumcised men most often get their HPV-associated lesions under the foreskin—remember how we said that HPV loves hot, moist areas? Circumcised men tend to get their lesions on the distal shaft of the penis (close to the head of the penis).

However, regardless of whether the man is circumcised or not, HPV can infect the skin at the base of the penis (typically not covered by a condom), the skin on the scrotum, or the skin lining the urethra. Unless these infections lead to bumps, bleeding, or itching, in most cases, men don't even know that they're carrying HPV or that they might be infectious. And even if they're being diligent and always wear condoms, condoms don't cover all of the potentially infected skin. Since HPV is spread by skin-to-skin

contact, this means that condoms cannot completely eliminate the risk of transmission to a female partner.

In general, men present fewer symptoms and serious
complications of HPV infection than do women. While penile cancer does occur, it's rare, at least in this country. Why
does HPV infection cause so much more mischief in the
cervical mucosa than on the penis? We don't really know,
but there are several possibilities. One is that HPV prefers
the local environment of the cervix better—there's lots of
stuff going on compared to the somewhat dry environment
of the penis. Another is that HPV may be affected by
women's menstrual cycling.

For all of these reasons, HPV infection of the penis is
not on the radar screen of most men, and neither is it on
the radar screen of most doctors. When men *do* go to the
doctor, they may not be examined for HPV infection. While
Pap smears are a regular part of women's exams, a man
may have to specifically request testing to rule out an HPV-
associated lesion. Since HPV testing is not available for
men, that leaves an examination of the penis as the only
way to make a diagnosis.

Many doctors can diagnose a wart on the penis, but
many—if not most—HPV infections on the penis are *subclinical.* This means that without training and specialized examination techniques, a doctor will miss most penile lesions. By
now you've probably already guessed what needs to be done:
examination of the penis with vinegar and magnification, just
as in the cervix. This is a technique that most doctors don't
know how to do, and in fact, the American Medical Association recommends against using it for screening purposes.

Why? Intuitively, it makes sense to do something about

lesions on the penis and reduce the risk of transmission to an uninfected partner, but there are no data suggesting that treating these lesions has any impact. The problem isn't that this approach wouldn't work; it's simply that we don't know that it would. And in the absence of knowing, the approach is to do nothing (similar to what is now done in the anal canal with anal screening).

The problems with penile screening are very real: Whom do we screen with penile examination? How often? Another problem with screening gets back to the training issue. While application of the vinegar definitely helps us see subtle lesions we'd otherwise miss, thereby increasing the sensitivity of the test, it's also rather nonspecific; lots of things cause acetowhitening that have nothing to do with HPV. On the penis, anything that causes any kind of irritation of the penile skin could cause acetowhitening—anything from penile warts to candida infection to having just gone for a good jog. Unless the doctor knows how to distinguish HPV-associated acetowhitening from the non-HPV-associated acetowhitening, many men might be overtreated, or even treated for a disease that they don't have.

If one approaches this problem from a public health perspective, it would *seem* to make sense to screen male partners of women with known HPV-associated genital disease. The idea would be to ask the male partners to come in for a penile examination, and to have clinical or subclinical disease treated. Some have argued against this approach, citing data that shows that treating the husbands of women who are being treated for dysplasia doesn't affect the disease recurrence rate in those women. They argue that the horse is already out of the barn, and that the HPV has already been spread between the partners.

Maybe. But it might be possible to infect areas of a partner's genital epithelium that aren't currently infected. And one could argue that there's the potential to prevent transmission to another partner who has never been infected. Today's monogamous relationship may not be so tomorrow.

In my practice, I prefer to examine male partners and treat their disease if it's detected. If a woman is diagnosed with an HPV-associated lesion, I usually ask her to bring in her partner, too, for an examination. The goal of the examination and treatment of the partner isn't to prevent penile cancer, but to lower the amount of infectious virus, since as in the cervix, most mature infectious viral particles live in lesions rather than in clinically normal-looking skin. As with everyone else, I have no evidence that this has any impact at all. This idea is very controversial; some doctors agree with me, while others don't. But to me, it seems like common sense.

In my experience, about half of all male partners of women with active genital disease will have some sign of HPV infection on the penis. It's interesting to speculate on the other half. Did he have a lesion in the past that resolved spontaneously after transmitting HPV to his partner? Or is the active genital disease in the woman due to an HPV type that she had before this partner, and that he either got infected but never developed the disease, or he never got infected at all? In most ways, the discussion is moot. We should focus on treating disease where we can find it, not on who gave what to whom. Not only is it usually irrelevant, but it's *impossible* to determine with any certainty.

Penile Examination

How is the penis examined? A diagram of the penis is shown in figure 14.1. First, I ask the man if he thinks he has anything. You'd be amazed how often men don't really know—or don't want to know—what's going on down below. I ask them to drop their pants and underwear and then paint vinegar—5 percent acetic acid—on the penis with a large swab. I also put acetic acid on the scrotum.

After a few minutes, I'll ask him to stand in front of a colposcope (yes, that ubiquitous colposcope), so that I can examine the penis under magnification. We don't absolutely have to use a colposcope for magnification—a good, strong magnifying glass will do.

The first place I examine is the opening of the urethra, the tube leading from the bladder to the outside of the penis. Examination of the end of the urethra is simply done by gently tugging on the opening of the very tip of the penis. About 15 percent of all men who have HPV infection on the penis will have it in the urethra. Fortunately, most of the time, the lesions are found in the last half centimeter or so, the visible area. Using this technique, a doctor can't see lesions that are higher up in the urethra; to examine that area, the doctor must use a small scope called a urethroscope. I refer patients for this somewhat unpleasant procedure only rarely—for instance, if someone has difficulty urinating, if he notes bleeding, or if the lesions in the visible part of the urethra do not resolve despite several attempts at therapy. While examining the urethra, I take care to avoid getting acetic acid near it—seepage of acetic acid into the urethra is not fun.

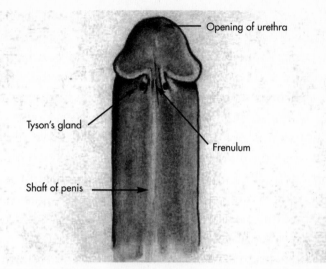

Opening of urethra

Tyson's gland

Frenulum

Shaft of penis

Figure 14.1: Diagram of the Penis. *This diagram shows the underside of the shaft of the penis. In the center is the frenulum, a piece of tissue that extends to the head of the penis. On either side of the frenulum is a small bump known as Tyson's glands. Like pearly penile papules (fig. 14.2), these can be mistaken for warts but are a normal part of the anatomy of the penis. (Illustration by Ira C. Smith.)*

After looking at the distal urethra, I methodically examine the entire skin surface of the penis and scrotum, looking for signs of subclinical infection on the penis as well as more obvious clinical disease (see below). Subclinical lesions do not occur with latent HPV infections: They reflect *active* infections, and while they may not be as infectious as clinically obvious, exophytic lesions, they should be treated with the same care and caution.

Distinguishing real HPV-associated lesions from normal variations of penile anatomy is important. Bumps that can be confused with true HPV-associated penile disease include a wonderfully named variant of normal anatomy called *pearly penile papules*. These are shown in figure 14.2. They're typically found in large numbers on the head of the penis nearest to the shaft (called the *corona*), and occasionally a few stragglers can be found on the shaft itself. *Condylomata latum*, a condition caused by secondary syphilis, can also be mistaken for genital warts. In this case, a penile exam is not enough, and a simple blood test can rule out or confirm syphilis. Also, you may find two bumps, one on each side of the frenulum. The frenulum is the little piece of tissue on the underside of the penis, in the middle, near the head, running parallel to the shaft (see fig. 14.1). These are called *Tyson's glands* and are *not* warts. Lots of other normal bumps, nooks, and crannies form the natural surface of a penis, and they can confuse the inexperienced doctor. Not only is treating these things as real lesions painful and pointless, but they don't go away even after multiple attempts to eradicate them. Only the patient goes away.

Occasionally, I perform a biopsy of the penile lesion, but most of the time it isn't necessary. The usual reasons to perform a biopsy are to diagnose subtle lesions where it isn't clear if they're related to HPV or not, and the patient really wants to know. Another reason is to rule out penile dysplasia. So far, you've heard about cervical dysplasia (CIN), vaginal dysplasia (VAIN), vulvar dysplasia (VIN), and anal dysplasia (AIN). A similar lesion occurs on the penis, and while we call it penile intraepithelial neoplasia, we don't abbreviate it as PIN, since that term is used for prostate disease. As with the other body parts, I'll refer to it as penile dysplasia here.

After I've finished examining the penis, I do a visual in-

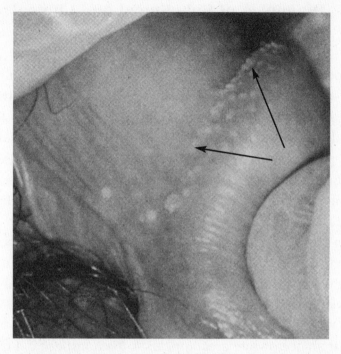

Figure 14.2: Pearly Penile Papules. *This photo shows pearly penile papules. These are bumps that typically appear in carpets on the head of the penis (see arrows) and occasionally spill out onto the penile shaft. Like Tyson's glands (fig. 14.1), these can be mistaken for warts but are a normal part of the anatomy of the penis. (Reprinted by permission of W. B. Saunders Company, Philadelphia, PA 19106. This illustration originally appeared in Palefsky, J. M. and R. Barrasso,* HPV Infection and Disease in Men, Obstetrics and Gynecology Clinics of North America, Human Papillomavirus II, *1996.)*

spection of the perianal region to look for warts, since this can be an area that HPV can infect. Because of the low likelihood of lesions inside the anal canal in heterosexual men, I don't usually perform an exam of the anal canal unless I see something perianally, or unless the man notes symptoms of intra-anal disease.

Diagnosis of Subclinical and Clinical Disease on the Penis

Some penile lesions grow exophytically, meaning that they cause bumps, and these are called clinical lesions. Subclinical lesions are flat. Most doctors are only trained to look for the clinical lesions. Once again the situation is similar to what I've described for HRA: The least dangerous disease is the most visible. If a man has obvious clinical disease, chances are that it's a condyloma that probably has HPV 6 or 11 in it—the types that can cause warts in women, but won't cause fatal disease. On the other hand, most doctors don't look for subclinical lesions. These lesions are more likely to contain oncogenic HPV types, the kinds that can cause fatal disease in women.

Makes you think, doesn't it?

If an acetowhite area appears to be nonspecific, I try to address the cause before deciding whether or not the patient also has an HPV-specific lesion. Some acetowhitening can be caused by yeast infection, and if I'm suspicious of that, I'll treat the patient with an antifungal cream and ask him to return for another exam in a few weeks. If there appears to be nonspecific inflammation that may be obscuring a real lesion, I'll give a 1 percent hydrocortisone cream for one to two weeks. Acetowhitening could also be due to psoriasis or lichen planus (a dark lesion, often purple, that can appear on the genitals; it's itchy and usually goes away with steroid cream). Giving hydrocortisone to someone with HPV infection could be locally immunosuppressive (that's bad for lesions caused by HPV), but it's safe for a

limited period of time and helps to determine if there's underlying HPV-related disease.

If a male has no signs of penile disease whatsover, he
should learn to examine himself. The analogy that I use
here is that of a cruise missile. A cruise missile has in its
electronic brain a detailed image of the terrain that it needs
to pass over to reach its programmed target. If a man mem-
orizes the terrain of his penis, since everything that he sees
at this point is normal, if and when something new crops
up, he's more likely to recognize it. This is the same philosophy as when your doctor tells you to memorize the
contours of your breast every month. On the penis, some
bumps appear suddenly and then they disappear almost as
quickly. More often than not, these are blocked oil glands.
HPV-related disease usually appears gradually and doesn't
go away quickly. I don't want men or their partners to get
crazy over this. A self-examination once every month or
two is probably sufficient, and it might be a good idea to
combine with a testicular self-examination. The woman, in
turn, could do her breast and genital self-examinations.
(Check appendices B and C for self-exam guidelines.)

Diagnosis of Penile Lesions

If evidence of clinical or subclinical infection is found, his
doctor may also want to perform a biopsy to rule out penile cancer or penile dysplasia (potentially precancerous
changes in the skin of the penis similar to those seen in the
cervix). Both of these conditions usually affect older patients, although penile dysplasia has become more com-

mon in recent years due to the widespread infection of HPV, with some help from HIV. If the doctor determines that there is no real danger of penile dysplasia or cancer, then the biopsy is largely unnecessary.

A punch biopsy is one way to obtain a penile sample, and is a fairly simple outpatient procedure. The area is anesthetized, and a Keyes punch (an instrument used to take a small round skin biopsy) removes a round specimen of skin at the site of the lesion. I send the biopsy to a pathologist for examination and cauterize or suture the biopsy area.

Another way to obtain a biopsy is to anesthetize the skin and remove the lesion with a forceps and scissors. Overall, the procedure is minimally painful; the worst part is the injection of lidocaine to freeze the lesion. Sometimes applying a topical lidocaine cream or spray lessens the pain of the lidocaine injection. (Certainly, the patient may suffer plenty of psychological discomfort.)

After the biopsy is done, the area may be a little sore, but it usually heals quickly and with minimal discomfort. Sometimes scarring may occur at the biopsy site.

What about HPV Detection Tests for Men?

Remember that I said collecting samples from penile skin for HPV testing is difficult. Detection of HPV in urine or sperm is also tough, especially in men without lesions. In fact, it's likely that the HPV detected in urine or sperm came from cells shed from lesions within the urethra. In addition, the act of masturbating to provide a sperm sample could cause shedding of cells from penile lesions. HPV DNA type can be determined with a biopsy, but there is usually no good reason to obtain this information from a clinical standpoint—it won't change the way the doctor manages either his male patient or the patient's partner(s).

Basically, the best method of detecting HPV is to look for the lesions that it causes, using a visual examination: a 5 percent acetic acid, a bright light, and a magnifying lens. Lesions can be identified through self-examination as well, although a doctor provides the best confirmation.

Penile Warts

We've already seen that high-risk male HPV infection can come in several different forms: subclinical disease, including penile dysplasia and clinical disease, often in the form of warts, also known as condyloma acuminatum.

Condyloma acuminata, or warts on the penis, are the whitish warts that resemble warts on other areas of the body. Their number can range from one to fifty. They can be confluent (blend together) and cover large areas of the genitalia. Penile condyloma often develop on areas most subjected to trauma during intercourse, and their appearance and treatment depend on their location. A photo of a penile wart is shown in figure 14.3.

In uncircumcised men, condyloma frequently appear on the inside of the prepuce (foreskin), at the frenulum, and on the head of the penis, while circumcised men usually develop warts on the shaft. Men may also develop warts on the inside of the urethra and in the urinary meatus, and

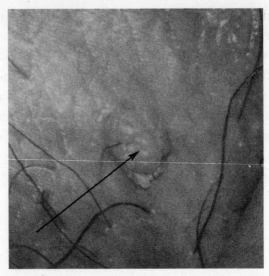

Figure 14.3: Penile Wart. *This photo shows a wart (condyloma acuminatum) on the penis (see arrow). (Reprinted by permission of W. B. Saunders Company, Philadelphia, PA 19106. This illustration originally appeared in Palefsky, J. M. and R. Barrasso,* HPV Infection and Disease in Men, Obstetrics and Gynecology Clinics of North America, Human Papillomavirus II, *1996.)*

this can obstruct urination. Men develop warts any time from three weeks to eight months after contact with the virus; in most men, the incubation period is about three months.

Appearance

The appearance of penile warts depends on their location. Mucosal warts that form around the urethra may be white or pink or red and have papillae (fingerlike projections). Heavily keratinized warts—the tougher, white warts that grow on drier skin—grow on the shaft of the penis and surrounding pubic area.

Penile intraepithelial neoplasia, or penile dysplasia, may be mistaken for genital warts, as could secondary syphilis and a host of normal lumps and bumps as described previously. Although both penile dysplasia and genital warts are caused by HPV, penile dysplasia indicates the presence of oncogenic HPV, which can, in rare cases, lead to penile cancer. High-risk HPV may also spread to the perineum or anus, causing anal dysplasia.

Treatment of Penile Warts

Depending on the size, number, and location of the warts, as well as the patient's desires, most physicians opt for topical treatment at first. Podofilox or imiquimod are both excellent choices. If the lesions persist after local treatment, then surgery is a good alternative. Topical and surgical treatments were covered in the previous chapter. Any patient, regardless of therapy, should see his doctor after the final treatment and every three months or so for a year (as long as the disease doesn't recur). Warts at the tip of the urethra can be treated with a dilute solution of 5-fluorouracil, TCA, or cryotherapy.

Recurrence

Within six months of treatment, about 10 percent to 20 percent of patients experience recurrent lesions. If your partner experiences recurrence, he and his physician can decide together if he should seek a different type of therapy. A biopsy of persistent condyloma should be considered if it resists repeated attempts at therapy. In the meantime, use condoms to prevent HPV transmission or reinfection.

Immunity heavily influences the frequency and severity of genital warts, and HIV-positive patients often experience more widespread, persistent infection. Whether or not HIV is a factor, improving general health—not smoking, better nutrition—can reduce the severity of infection. Despite this generally wholesome advice, even the healthiest of men may experience difficulty treating their penile warts, as well as frustrating recurrences.

Penile Dysplasia

About one half of penile dysplasia cases are subclinical. That means *one half* of men with active HPV infections show no outward symptoms without the assistance of acetic acid and colposcopic examinations.

Penile dysplasia is an unusual condition in the United States; it's more common among older men and among uncircumcised men. In the United States, circumcision is practiced more routinely, and HPV has a smaller chance of taking hold in the circumcised penis. European men have a higher incidence of penile dysplasia; uncircumcised men are three times more likely to develop penile dysplasia. In addition, subclinical disease is less common among circumcised men, since these infections are most often localized to the prepuce, or foreskin.

The term *bowenoid papulosis* was coined in 1978 to describe inconspicuous lesions that show some characteristics of severe penile dysplasia, or squamous cell carcinoma in situ. They are often flat or slightly elevated, red or brown lesions with a smooth, glistening surface. A photo of Bowenoid papulosis is shown in figure 14.4. Acetowhitening reactions are strong in these areas, and the pattern of blood vessels in the whitened area is similar to that of severe dysplasia.

The course of penile dysplasia is usually chronic, with an average duration of two to three years. Lesions often regress spontaneously, and penile dysplasia is generally regarded as benign and self-limited, especially in younger men. Older patients, though, need to be observed closely, especially if the lesion persists or spreads to other genital areas.

These lesions probably carry infectious virus, though probably less than in the florid warts that were covered earlier in this chapter. Men who are lesion-free (latent) are not likely to be infectious, but HPV can reactivate at any time. Immunosuppression (HIV infection, for example) is the most common reason for HPV reactivation, especially among men who have sex with men (MSM).

Treatment of Penile Dysplasia

If subclinical HPV infection *is* confirmed through acetowhitening, many physicians opt for the wait-and-see method of treatment. Often the lesion goes away by itself. In clinically normal penile skin, HPV probably isn't infectious or is at least poorly infectious. With either subclinical or clinical lesions, though, a man *is* infectious and should take appropriate measures to minimize the risk of transmission to a sexual partner and to avoid spreading HPV to other parts of the anogenital epithelium. At a minimum that

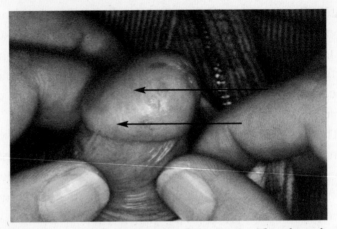

Figure 14.4: Bowenoid Papulosis of the Penis. *This photo shows Bowenoid papules on the head of the penis (see arrows). These are typically red or brown and can be found anywhere on the penis. When biopsied they show moderate or severe dysplasia of the penis. These lesions have the potential to progress to cancer of the penis and should be treated. (Photo courtesy of Dr. Timothy Berger, University of California, San Francisco.)*

means no shaving of the pubic hair or hair around the opening of the anus. It also means that a man should avoid scratching down there.

If a penile dysplasia lesion persists, a physician may remove it with laser vaporization or electrosurgery. These lesions can also be treated with TCA and liquid nitrogen. Treatment with podofilox or imiquimod isn't currently recommended, as the Food and Drug Administration has only approved these for treatment of genital warts. If invasive cancer is suspected, wide local excision usually removes all of the cancer. Penile cancer, though, is extremely rare, and only develops in a small percentage of cases.

Risk Factors

The risk factors for penile dysplasia are largely based on the risk factors for HPV infection and vary only slightly from cervical cancer risks. Sex at an early age, while not physically damaging to men, usually indicates an increased number of sexual partners. In addition, compromised immunity, either related to smoking or HIV infection, can increase the severity of HPV infection.

Risk Factors for Penile Dysplasia

- **HPV infection.** HPV infection is often the direct cause of penile dysplasia.
- **History of sexually transmitted diseases.** Other STDs can weaken the penis's immunity and allow penile dysplasia to develop more quickly.
- **Lowered immunity due to HIV and other conditions.** HIV is the most common immunity disorder related to penile dysplasia, but other circumstances, such as recent organ transplant, can allow HPV to take hold.
- **Smoking.** Smoking cigarettes causes cancer and lowers your immunity. Nicotine is also a contributing factor to impotence. Another good reason to quit.
- **Uncircumcised penis.** Studies have shown that uncircumcised men have an increased risk of penile dysplasia, penile cancer, and persistent HPV infection; the virus often takes hold in the foreskin. Poor hygiene under the foreskin is one of the strongest risk factors.
- **Poor general health.** Poor nutrition and general health lowers your body's general immunity.
- **Poor health care.** Regular visits to a physician can catch penile dysplasia in the earlier stages.

Penile Cancer

In extremely rare cases in the United States, penile dysplasia can progress to invasive penile cancer. Penile cancer accounts for about 0.2 percent of all cancers in men, and occurs in about 1 per 100,000 men per year. Most men in the United States are circumcised at birth, and as we know, that cuts back the risk of developing penile dysplasia. Even if a man does develop penile dysplasia, it's usually fairly harmless, requiring only vigilance and regular exams.

That said, penile cancer does occur more commonly in developing countries—in some countries in South America and Africa, penile cancer makes up 10 percent of all cases of cancer in men! Like cervical cancer, it's usually linked to HPV infection—so it's worth outlining in this chapter. Not surprisingly, there's a link between cervical and penile cancer in married couples.

Symptoms

Symptoms of penile cancer include growths or sores on the penis, any abnormal discharge or liquid coming from the penis, pain, or bleeding. If a man experiences any of these symptoms, he should see his doctor immediately for a thorough exam, which will probably include colposcopic examination and biopsy.

Staging and Treatment of Penile Cancer

If the biopsy confirms the presence of cancerous cells, then the patient will begin staging. (The methods for staging are covered on pages 151–156.)

Penile cancer includes the following stages.

Stage	What It Means
I	Cancer cells are found only on the surface of the glans (the head) and on the foreskin.
II	Cancer cells are found in the deeper tissues of the glans and have spread to the shaft of the penis.
III	Cancer is found in the penis and has spread to nearby lymph nodes in the groin.
IV	Cancer cells are found throughout the penis and the lymph nodes in the groin and/or have spread to other parts of the body.
Recurrent	The cancer has come back, in the penis or elsewhere, after treatment.

Treatment

As with all cancers, penile cancer is treated by stage, type, the patient's age and overall condition. Clinical trials are available at every stage.

Stage I

Because the cancer is localized, Stage I has a terrific cure rate. If the cancer is limited to the foreskin, treatment will likely be wide local excision and circumcision. If the cancer begins in the glans and doesn't involve other tissues, treatment may involve fluorouracil cream and microsurgery (removal of the cancer). If the tumor begins in the glans and involves other tissues, treatment may involve partial penectomy (amputation of the penis) and lymph node removal; external radiation therapy; and microsurgery.

Stage II

In Stage II, cancer cells have spread to the glans and shaft of the penis, and surgery is usually the best route: partial, total, or radical penectomy, or radiation therapy followed by penectomy. Clinical trials on laser therapy for penile cancer are also in progress.

Stage III

Stage III involves cancer that has spread beyond the penis, so in addition to penectomy, lymph node removal on both sides of the groin, radiation therapy and chemotherapy may also be required. A variety of different chemotherapy drugs have been used in penile cancer in combination with radiation therapy, including vincristine, bleomycin, and methotrexate. Cisplatin in combination with 5-fluorouracil has also been used. The side effects of cisplatin and 5-fluorouracil were covered in chapters 7 and 8, respectively. The most common side effects of vincristine are abdominal cramps and numbness and tingling of the hands and feet; side effects of bleomycin include fever, chills, loss of appetite, sores in the mouth, and changes in the nails; and methotrexate can cause damage to the bone marrow, sores in the mouth with changed taste, diarrhea, skin changes, and kidney damage. All are associated with decreased fertility.

Stage IV

Because the cancer has spread to other parts of the body, Stage IV prognosis is not good; at this point, clinical trials should be strongly considered and chemotherapy and radiation therapy may be used for palliative purposes to lessen the symptoms. Penectomy, wide local excision, and microsurgery are also likely treatments.

Recurrent Penile Cancer

If the penile cancer has come back, amputation of the penis, radiation therapy, and chemotherapy clinical trials can offer symptom relief.

Treatment Options for Penile Cancer

Microsurgery

Microsurgery of the penis is a common treatment for localized cancer. It removes *only* the cancer, and as little normal tissue as possible; microsurgery also provides a biopsy for study by a pathologist. The doctor will likely use a microscope to confirm removal of all cancerous cells.

Circumcision

Circumcision, commonly performed immediately after birth, can also be done in adult men (although it usually requires more healing time). Circumcision is a relatively simple procedure, removes only the foreskin, and provides a biopsy for study.

Penectomy, or Amputation of the Penis

While it may seem drastic, amputation of the penis is the most common and most effective treatment of penile cancer. In a partial penectomy, only part of the penis is taken out; in a total penectomy, the whole penis is removed. A surgeon may also choose to remove lymph nodes in the groin during this surgery.

Other Options

Radiation therapy, chemotherapy, clinical trials, and wide local excision are covered in earlier chapters in detail.

Anal HPV Infection and Anal Dysplasia in Men

In chapter 10 I discussed the various issues surrounding anal HPV infection, anal dysplasia, and anal cancer in women. Of course, men have behinds, too, and the very same issues apply to men. So I'll ask you to refer to that chapter for the details.

Of course, a few subtle differences exist. Of all the

groups studied so far, we know the most about anal HPV infection and anal dysplasia among men who have sex with men (MSM). We know the least about anal HPV infection and anal dysplasia in men who have never had receptive anal intercourse. We do, however, know that men who've never had receptive anal intercourse can get anal HPV infection. As I indicated earlier, it's not that uncommon for male partners of women to have perianal warts. How did they get there? Again, we get back to the same risk factors—fingers, toys, and even "auto-inoculation," or spreading the infection from other parts of a person's own genitals by scratching or shaving, etc. HPV could even migrate up, causing intra-anal lesions.

As I indicated earlier, I routinely check for perianal lesions in men who have never had receptive anal intercourse if they're referred to me for assessment of penile disease. If I see a perianal wart, then I'll treat it as described in chapter 10. If the wart doesn't respond to therapy, I'll do HRA to rule out an internal lesion.

Anal HPV infection in MSM is a whole other ball of wax. Several studies, including a few of my own, have been performed in this group of men. This group has been intensively studied because the relatively high number of partners with whom they have receptive anal intercourse, as well as the frequency of receptive anal intercourse, puts them at higher risk. The high incidence of HIV infection in this group throws another wrinkle into the equation: HPV infection and its lesions are more severe in immunocompromised individuals.

Basically, my group and others have shown the following: Anal HPV infection is very common (found in more than 60 percent of HIV-negative MSM and more than 90 percent of HIV-positive MSM). HIV-positive MSM have a higher number of anal HPV types, higher prevalence of anal dysplasia, and higher rate of development of moderate and severe anal dysplasia than HIV-negative MSM. Each of these items correlated with the level of T-helper lymphocytes, also known as the CD4 level. T-helper or CD4 lymphocytes help to fight infection, and damage to the body's ability to ward off viruses such as HPV occurs when HIV destroys these lymphocytes. The lower the CD4 level, indicating more advanced immunosuppression, the higher the rate of anal HPV infection and anal dysplasia. As I mentioned earlier, the rate of anal cancer is high among HIV-negative MSM (about 35 per 100,000, versus about 8 per 100,000 for cervical cancer in the general population of women), but it's even higher among HIV-positive MSM. Current estimates are that the incidence of anal cancer among HIV-positive MSM is about twice that in HIV-negative MSM!

Whew. That's a lot of numbers. What I want to say is that among MSM, anal cancer is as common as cervical cancer was before the good Dr. Papanicolaou discovered the Pap smear. Put differently, anal cancer among both HIV-negative and HIV-positive MSM is *more* common than is cervical cancer in the general population of women.

You may also have heard that many individuals with HIV are showing substantial improvement due to a series of drugs collectively known as *highly active antiretroviral therapy,* or HAART. This includes the drugs known as *protease inhibitors.* Other infections due to opportunistic viruses (such as the virus that causes Kaposi's sarcoma) in

HIV-positive men and women appear to get better when these individuals start HAART, perhaps due to improvement in the immune system. The same does not appear to be true, however, for HPV-associated disease. While some researchers have shown some improvement in anogenital neoplasia after an individual starts HAART, the effect is modest at best.

This is an issue of some concern. As you may recall, I mentioned earlier that progression from high-grade neoplasia to invasive cancer may take many years. In the pre-HAART era, more HIV-positive men and women might have developed anal or cervical cancer had they not died first of their HIV disease; their high-grade cervical or anal dysplasia didn't have time to progress. Now, these individuals, thankfully, are living longer due to HAART. But if their severe dysplasia doesn't improve, with HAART, they may now have the time to progress to cancer, especially if we don't screen for these lesions and treat them. Bottom line: These wonderful HIV drugs may paradoxically lead to even higher rates of anal cancer in the near future. Stay tuned as we look at this carefully over the next few years.

So what to do? If you're a male and have a history of receptive anal intercourse, you should be screened with an anal Pap smear, whether you're HIV-positive or HIV-negative. If you're HIV-negative, you should be screened every two to three years after the age of forty. If you're HIV-positive, you should be screened every year. If any of those Paps comes back positive, you'll need an HRA, with biopsy and treatment as described in chapter 10.

One concern may cross your mind: Can HIV-positive people tolerate all these procedures? The answer is yes—

they do very well indeed, and appear to be at no higher risk of complications than HIV-negative individuals. On the other hand, if someone is so sick with HIV that he is not expected to live for much longer, then these anal diagnostic procedures shouldn't be performed at all, since detection and treatment of anal dysplasia to prevent anal cancer isn't likely to be of much value. Fortunately, with HAART, situations such as this are becoming increasingly rare.

If you're a male who has never had receptive anal intercourse, you should consider having an anal Pap smear if you have a history of anal warts inside or outside the anal canal, if you have a history of anal bleeding, pain, or itching, bleeding with bowel movements, or if you think you have a growth inside the anal canal. Many of these symptoms can be found with hemorrhoids, but sometimes they can be due to anal dysplasia.

Conclusion

Although penile HPV infection is as common as female-associated HPV infection, it's far more difficult to detect without regular doctor visits. Usually, men will have to specifically request colposcopic examination, and if they don't know they have an HPV infection, they're not likely to do that. If you're a woman with HPV, you may want to suggest that your partner see a doctor to request at least the "vinegar" test.

Generally, penile HPV infection comes and goes on its own, and judging how infectious the virus is at any time is difficult. Clinical infection is the most infectious; subclinical infection is still infectious, although perhaps less so than clinical. If your partner exhibits absolutely no apparent infection, he's *probably* not infectious, although he may still be carrying a dormant HPV virus.

If your partner has penile dysplasia, then your partner's doctor is the best judge of treatment. Penile intraepithelial neoplasia rarely advances to penile cancer, and unless the patient is older or has an immunity disorder, the lesion will most likely go away on its own.

In the meantime, as long as your partner has signs of active HPV disease, be it clinical or subclinical, use condoms to help prevent HPV transmission and reinfection. As always, keep in mind that condoms do not cover all infectious areas, and transmission is still possible.

The natural history of HPV in men is an area that requires more research before we can make any absolute statements, but because women are more negatively affected by HPV infection, most of the research is focused on the prevention of cervical cancer development.

As I stated in chapter 1, choose your sexual partners carefully. With due vigilance, oncogenic HPV is a fairly harmless virus; monogamous couples usually just accept that if one of them has HPV, they'll both have it sooner or later. Knowing the risks and maintaining your general health will keep the virus—and the risk of cancer—at bay.

If you or your male partner has a history of receptive anal intercourse, you should consider having an anal Pap smear, especially if you or he has HIV infection. The name of the game here is prevention: If you have moderate or severe anal dysplasia, you're probably at risk of developing anal cancer. Detection and treatment of these anal lesions can probably prevent that from happening.

PART SIX

Taking Control

CHAPTER FIFTEEN

Living with HPV and Talking with Your Partner

Now you know the truth: HPV, on its own, won't kill you. But the bottom line is that HPV itself isn't curable; we can only treat the lesions that it causes. Close follow-up—frequent treatment of recurring warts and Pap smears regardless of HPV type—is the best *physical* therapy, but even that doesn't always help the emotional or mental trial of having an STD.

If you're like many of my patients, the idea of HPV is embarrassing or even shameful. STDs are so stigmatized in our society that the very thought of having one might make you feel dirty or somehow defective, as though you'll never be desirable as a person again. You might feel guilty or stupid because you didn't use a condom, or you might feel like you are being punished for having sex. Even if you're not plagued with the guilt issues, you may experience general health anxiety. On top of your personal anxieties, you may have to tell your partner, from whom you may or may not have acquired the virus, and think about what to tell future partners as well.

Here's a list of questions most HPV patients ask (or are afraid to ask) when they get the news:

Common Questions of People with HPV Infection

- Who infected me with the virus?
- When was I infected with the virus?
- If so many people have HPV, should I tell anyone? What should I tell my current partner?
- What should I tell my previous partners? Should I talk to *all* of them?
- What should I tell future partners?
- Will I have to use condoms forever?
- Will I ever be noninfectious?
- Should my current partner be examined too?
- Could my partner reinfect me?
- Is there any risk in having oral sex?
- Can oral-anal sex transmit HPV infection?
- How will my life change once I am told that I have HPV infection?
- How should I change my lifestyle?

Every one of these questions is equally important—and equally difficult to answer. I'll do my best to help answer each of them, but in the end, the decisions are yours to make.

Who Infected Me? And When?

I answered some of this way back in chapter 1 and a few other chapters. Generally, oncogenic HPV shows outward signs of infection within about three to four months. That's if it shows these signs at all, of course; HPV may stay dormant or latent for many months or even years before other factors trigger an active infection. Genital warts due to nononcogenic HPV types sometimes require less incubation time; a patient may show warts within four to six weeks after infection. So it's difficult to come up with a hard-and-fast rule. Bottom line: usually three to four months, but anything is possible.

So that answers when, which may help indicate *who*. If you've been in a monogamous relationship for over a year and only recently developed HPV-related disease, you may have gotten HPV before the relationship and had a latent infection. It may have had nothing to do with your current partner. But during the relationship, you may also have gotten HPV from your partner, who (1) may not have known that he had it from a previous relationship or (2) may have gotten it from another partner recently.

Because of the latency period, narrowing down these alternatives is virtually impossible, unless one of you had never engaged in sexual contact before the relationship. To put this in a different context, successfully suing for divorce on grounds of infidelity—based on HPV infection—would be very difficult.

If you're *not* in a monogamous relationship, and you've had multiple partners recently, the question of *who* is just as tricky. Again, latency periods can prevent you from ever knowing exactly when and who, but think about the most obvious questions first. Have you had unprotected sexual contact with anyone recently, or around the likely time of transmission? If you had unprotected sex with someone four months prior to your appointment—but protected sex in other cases—then the unprotected partner is a possible candidate, but still you can't be sure.

This may or may not help narrow down the question of who infected you, as well as any partners you may have infected. But perhaps the most important point to take home is that knowing with any real certainty is virtually impossible, and when all is said and done, it doesn't really matter. What *does* matter is that you, your partners, and anyone else at risk be examined for signs of HPV-related lesions.

What Should I Tell My Current Partner?

My advice is to be honest with him or her, as tough as that seems. Find out everything you need to know about your infection and how it might affect your partner. Tell him what you know, and what your treatments will be, and tell him how he might be affected by HPV. You might want to bring him along to your physician's office so she can answer any additional questions. You could also give him this book to read.

Assuming that you've just been diagnosed with dysplasia but you haven't yet been treated, and you're trying to figure out what to say to your partner, you could say something like:

"I just wanted to let you know that my doctor told me

that I have HPV, human papillomavirus. I haven't been treated, but I'll be treated soon. HPV is a very common sexually transmitted virus, and it's possible that I've already infected you with HPV, or that you were the person who gave me the HPV. We'll never know who gave it to who. It doesn't show up on blood tests, so you might want to ask your doctor to examine you for any signs of it."

If you haven't been using condoms with this partner, and you plan to have sex with him in the future, you could add:

"Until both of us have been 'certified' free of disease, we should probably use condoms. On the other hand, we've been having sex for a while without using condoms, and it may not make much sense for us to start now. Also, condoms probably lower the risk of spreading HPV, but they don't stop it completely. So it's a bit of a tough call. Once both of us have been treated and/or shown to be free of disease, there's still a chance that we could spread HPV to each other, but it's pretty small."

If you think that you may have given it to your partner, you may want to apologize. If you need to, then go for it, but keep in mind that you didn't know you had HPV at the time. Don't beat yourself up for it. If you used condoms, you can explain that the chances of transmission are less than if you hadn't, and again, let him know that standard blood tests don't test for HPV. Give him all the information he needs to know, and if he asks you questions you can't answer, tell him to buy this book or ask his doctor.

What Should I Tell a Previous Partner? Should I Talk to *All* of Them?

If you're reasonably sure who gave you HPV—or even if you think you may have had sex with him after your infection, in which case you may have given it to him—my advice is to give him a call. This is often even more difficult than telling a current partner; after all, it's possible you may not see him anymore, or that you're not on speaking terms, or any of the things that can happen after a sexual relationship ends. Since HPV is such a dicey virus, it's tough to know if he gave it to or got it from you, but in any case, he's been exposed to it.

The question of how far back you need to go is a tough one, and once again you'll need to use your own judgment. If you've recently been diagnosed with dysplasia, it probably doesn't make sense to go back to partners that you had a very long time ago. My suggestion—based on no data at all—would be to cut it off at about two years.

If you do have a way to get in touch with a previous partner and you feel that you should tell him, though, swallow the lump in your throat and just go for it. You'll feel much better for letting him know—after all, he may be spreading the disease without knowing it—and he'll be able to ask his doctor for the vinegar test. You don't have to accuse him; just give him the information you have.

Here's a possible way to start the conversation:

"Hi. I just wanted to let you know that my doctor told me that I have HPV, human papillomavirus, and it's possible that I got it around the time that we slept together. It's also possible that I gave it to you. It's a very common sexually transmitted virus, and it doesn't show up on blood tests, so you might want to ask your doctor to examine you for any signs of it."

That's it. He may say it wasn't him, or that he's already been tested, or any of the other denials people make in difficult situations. (Think about how you felt in the doctor's office. Your first reaction was probably, "Not me!") Try not to take any offense to anything he says; he's probably as upset as you were when you found out. Just try to encourage him to go to his doctor for the vinegar test, and make it clear that regular blood tests—the type that test for HIV and syphilis—do *not* detect HPV. Let him know, too, that he might have imperceptible symptoms; he might believe that if he doesn't have a visible wart, he doesn't have HPV.

A conversation like this can be emotionally trying for both you and your former partner, so I advise telling him only after (1) you're sure you have signs of HPV infection, and (2) you've had some time to get used to the idea yourself. Calling him minutes after finding out will likely result in accusations and arguments, and at that point, you probably won't have all the information you need for yourself, much less someone else. Don't wait too long—keep in mind that other women are at risk for infection—but call him once you've taken some deep breaths and know what you'll tell him. Remember—you'll feel better for having told him, and he'll be able to find out if he has any active infection. In addition, he'll be able to tell his future partners that they might be exposed to HPV.

As with your current partner, give him all the information he needs to know, and if he asks you questions you can't answer, tell him to buy this book or ask his doctor.

And as I said before, you may want to wait to have this conversation until you've given yourself some time to think it over.

What Should I Tell Future Partners?

Moving on to another tough conversation: telling future partners. It's difficult, no question. After all, you at least have some level of intimacy with your past partners; although telling them is difficult, you have a starting point for a conversation.

With a new partner, though, you may have met them only recently. What if you tell him, and he rejects you? What if the news scares him away? If you tell him, and he decides not to be with you, then he's confirming what you already suspected: Having HPV makes you unlovable.

Often after getting an STD—especially a virus that can't be cured—patients develop a fear of intimacy. You could be afraid of getting another virus or of giving the virus to someone; and, worst of all, what if no one wants you because of HPV?

The simple truth is that HPV does *not* change who you are as a person. It alters you physically, of course, and the experience of having an STD may change the way you look at relationships and sex.

Not telling him is an option, but, plainly put, in my opinion it's a bad option. Try thinking about the situation from his perspective. If the person who infected you had known he had it, wouldn't you have wanted to have the option of saying yes or no with that information? Maybe you would have decided it wasn't worth it.

On the other hand, if he had been someone you wanted to develop a relationship with—or someone who was worth the risk of an STD—maybe you would have had sex anyway. But you would have done so with full knowledge of the risks and you probably would have used protection.

Telling a prospective partner may feel like giving *him* the control: He has the power to decide what happens in your relationship. That can be a frightening feeling, especially if you're already convinced that having HPV makes you less worthy as a person. In reality, though, you're the one in control: You have the information and you know HPV is not a factor of who you are as a person. If he decides to end the relationship, that's his prerogative. And you can walk away knowing that you did the right thing in telling him.

More often, though, you'll probably find that it won't be the problem you anticipate. I'd imagine (and hope) that most sexually active people in the new millennium *expect* to use condoms. It used to be that you actively chose to wear a condom; now, it seems, you actively choose *not* to wear a condom. As long as he has all the information, and you're honest with him early on, he should appreciate and respect you more for telling him.

Here are a few things you could say:

"In the past I was diagnosed with a lesion that indicates that I have or had HPV infection. I've been treated, and it appears to be gone. The HPV infection is probably gone too, but it's also possible that I still have it. Right now, though, I don't have any active disease, so even if I do have HPV infection, my chances of giving it to you are very small. I just wanted you to know because there's a risk of transmitting HPV to you, however small. Using condoms can decrease this small risk even more. The other thing you should know is that, based on my reading, since HPV is such a common virus, you have a good chance of having been exposed to HPV yourself by one or more of your previous partners. Have you ever been checked?"

If So Many People Have HPV, Should I Tell Anyone at All?

Yes. That's the easiest question for me to answer. One of the reasons so many people have HPV is because so few people talk, or even *know*, about it. If your current, future, and past partners don't know they're at risk, then they'll continue infecting new partners, who won't know they're at risk, and the cycle spins on. Ultimately, the decision to tell is up to you, but imagine yourself in their place: Wouldn't you rather have known your partner had HPV? You may not have changed your mind, but you would have appreciated the information.

Ignorance will not stop an epidemic. Only awareness and education—and proper use of that education—will.

Will I Have to Use Condoms Forever?

This question is linked to the next question on the list: Will I ever be noninfectious? The answer is as complicated and tough as the question.

I've said that active disease—dysplasia, genital warts, etc.,—is the most infectious stage of HPV infection. I've also said that latent infection, in which HPV numbers are so low as to be untraceable, is most likely poorly infectious or not infectious at all. So, you may be infectious while you have an active lesion, and you are probably not very infectious in the absence of a detectable lesion.

Most women reach a point where HPV is not detectable, so their chances of being infectious are very, very low. As I've said, new partners should know you've been treated for it, but you can indicate that you're currently free of disease and that the risk of transmission is low. If he's concerned about transmission, he can certainly request examination from his doctor.

Some couples absolutely hate using condoms, and it ruins the sexual experience for one or both of them. Other couples don't want to use condoms because they're trying to have a baby. Basically, the condom question is between you and your partner. Most long-term monogamous partners—married couples, for instance—recognize that if one has HPV, eventually they'll both probably have HPV infection.

Most often, a couple comes to me after they've been having unprotected sex for years. In this case, recommending condom use seems almost silly. On the other hand, there's still a concern for reinfection or infection of new areas. Nothing is risk-free, of course, but I usually advise a couple to use condoms while one or both of them has an active lesion. Both partners will hopefully have sought medical attention for diagnosis and treatment of HPV-related lesions, and once both have been declared disease-free for at least three months, they can resume sex without condoms.

But the truth is, if a couple asks me what the data are—the benefits of condom use—I'd say we have very little information. In fact, the little information we have suggests that condoms provide little benefit in preventing spread of HPV between long-standing sexual partners. Once again, I return to that old standby: common sense. I do recognize, however, that other doctors may well come up with totally different recommendations.

If a couple chooses not to use condoms, that's not necessarily an irrational choice. As with anything in life, some risk is always involved, and one of the few nice things about HPV infection is that it creates no long-term serious health consequences as long as you have regular screenings. If you're in a relationship that may not be long-term, condoms are probably a good idea, anyway, to prevent transmission of all STDs.

Should My Current Partner Be Tested for HPV Too?

Although testing your partner is not a universal approach—most doctors would assume your partner has HPV (especially if you had sex during your active infection). They believe that since men rarely exhibit any serious long-term consequences of HPV infection, treatment probably isn't necessary. In my practice, though, I usually recommend that he come in for an exam. First of all, it'll confirm whether or not he has an active infection, subclinical or clinical, and he can decide if he wants to treat it. Secondly, if he knows he's contracted HPV, he can tell his future partners. My philosophy has always been the more you know, the better.

Could My Partner Reinfect Me?

Reinfection occurs when your partner, who has an active HPV infection, passes that infection back to you after your disease has been cleared and/or declared latent. This could occur if his active infection comes in contact with a new, uninfected area of your epithelium. In this case, it's not really considered reinfection, since the area is new. Moreover, that "reinfection" could represent spread from your own HPV-infected epithelium elsewhere in your genital tract.

Several factors can contribute to a recurrence, which is the return of the disease at the original site of infection. Genital warts recur frequently and often spread, and dysplasia can recur in certain situations.

Factors leading to a recurrence include both psychological and physical stress. I've often had a patient whom I haven't seen in years come in with a recurrence, and my first question is usually, "What's going on in your life?" Often something big and stressful is going on. (At one point, I had quite a few patients who were law students, and I always knew when the bar exams were coming up. I'd suddenly become very busy with them.)

Physical stress can play a role, too—anything that puts your anogenital epithelium under stress. Inflammation due to other infection-causing agents such as gonorrhea, chlamydia, yeast, and trichomonas could theoretically trigger a recurrence, as well as a new, irritating vaginal product such as a douche or spermicidal cream.

So what can you do? One obvious answer is to lower your stress level, which we both know is easier said than done. But determining if you have a vaginal or cervical infection, or changing some of the vaginal products that you use, should be easy enough, right?

If both you and your partner are free of any active infection, reinfection is relatively unlikely. Lesions carry the most infectious virus.

Is There Any Risk in Having Oral Sex?

This question comes up all the time. For instance, I may have just advised a couple to use condoms while one or both of them has a genital lesion, and the next question is: Can we have oral sex? The answer to the question is a qualified yes.

Having oral sex with someone with a genital lesion *could* lead to HPV transmission to the mouth. This probably does happen, but rarely. Having said that, HPV infection in the mouth isn't that uncommon. Some HPV types, such as HPV 13 and 32, live primarily in the mouth and rarely live elsewhere. But the mouth *can* sometimes contain genital HPV types such as 6, 11, 16, or 18, presumably acquired through oral sex with an infected partner.

What are the consequences of oral HPV infection? The vast majority of the time, none at all, and that's why I tell partners that they're unlikely to run into trouble. Rarely, though, a person can develop oral warts or, even more rarely, oral cancer, for all the same reasons that HPV can cause anogenital cancer. While HPV is definitely associated with oral cancer, the association isn't nearly as strong as in the cervix or anus, where almost *all* cancers are associated with HPV. Only a fraction of oral cancers are associated with HPV, perhaps up to 30 percent (the numbers vary from study to study), and some types of oral cancer are more likely to contain HPV than others. Oddly, one of the oral cancers most strongly associated with HPV is cancer of the tonsils!

So yes, HPV can cause problems in the mouth, and this can be the result of oral sex. Oral warts can be painful and difficult to treat, often with surgical excision, liquid nitrogen, and podophyllin. Oral cancer can be fatal. However, oral sex is an integral part of the sexual relationship of many couples, and after I've explained the risks, most opt to continue to have it, a decision that makes sense to me. On the other hand, it's also perfectly reasonable to abstain from oral sex until the partner who is playing the passive role in the oral sex act has been shown to be free of disease.

Can Oral-Anal Sex Transmit HPV Infection?

We don't really know, since we don't have enough data. But common sense dictates that it probably can, for all of the same reasons that oral-genital sex can.

How Will My Life Change Once I Am Told That I Have HPV Infection?

If you have cervical HPV, your physical life should change very little. After you and your doctor decide on a treatment—waiting, LEEP, or whatever may be appropriate to your case—that's it. You'll have to return for your follow-up Paps, of course, and consider all of the above questions about informing your partners. Physically, however, you should be healthy after your treatment.

Genital warts, on the other hand, may require more maintenance. The treatments often last several weeks or even months, and you may have to return to your doctor's office for frequent checkups. In addition, genital warts carry a higher rate of recurrence, so you'll have to keep a closer watch on their development.

Support groups are available online for all HPV patients—cervical, genital warts, and cancer—and you can check appendix D for resources.

How *Should* I Change My Lifestyle?

This is the part where I advise you, give you general doctor's orders—and it's up to you to follow them.

First of all, I can't stress enough the fact that good general health can help prevent, or at least lessen the severity of, recurrent dysplasia and genital warts. It remains a fact, though, that even people who take incredibly good care of themselves can still suffer the consequences of HPV infection.

Quit smoking! Quit smoking whenever possible, or at least reduce your nicotine intake. It doesn't take a medical degree to understand reports attesting to the deadly carcinogens in a cigarette. If the threats of lung cancer and emphysema aren't enough, the double threat of HPV and smoking increases your risk for any kind of anogenital dysplasia or cancer.

Improve your nutrition. Better nutrition contributes to your immunity and could lessen the severity and frequency of disease. Women with diets high in vegetables, fruits, carotenoids, and vitamins C and E may be at lower risk of developing cervical cancer. If for some reason you are unable to eat a complete, well-balanced diet, you should consider taking folic acid and vitamin A supplements.

Get your Pap smears! I know, I know, if I've said it once, I've said it a thousand times. Just like you've heard that smoking causes cancer, you've heard that early detection is the key to curing cancer. Pap smears are our best method of detecting cancerous changes in your cervix. Attend your three- and six-month follow-ups, and get your annual pelvic exam. While you're at it, consider getting an HIV blood test.

Use condoms. Although condoms aren't 100 percent effective against HPV, they can decrease the risk of transmission. In addition, they protect against other STDs, including HIV, not to mention pregnancy, and even help reduce urinary tract infections and yeast infections.

Be selective about your sexual partners. Communicate with your partners before you decide to engage in sexual activity. You've already experienced the pain of finding out you have an STD and are dealing with the consequences. On the grand scale of STDs, HPV should be one of the more harmless: With proper medical care, it won't kill you, and except for some cases of genital warts, rarely recurs. But dozens of other diseases—HIV, herpes, and syphilis, to name a few—have far-reaching, even fatal, consequences.

Fewer sexual partners lead to fewer chances for transmitting an STD (although, as we know, it only takes one partner to transmit HPV). Communicating with your partners leads to more informed choices and, often, a more fulfilling sexual life.

Conclusion

I hope this chapter has helped to answer some of the more difficult HPV-related issues. As a doctor, I can give you all the medical and scientific information you want (and maybe some you don't), but using that information is entirely up to you. The stigma attached to having an STD is considerable, and as I mentioned earlier, you may be experiencing feelings of shame, anger, guilt, or depression. They're all normal reactions.

Now that you know the facts about HPV, though, you have real information you can use in your present and future. You can never go into the past and "un-get" HPV, but you have complete control of your own future. Learn as much as you can, use that information wisely, and take control!

PART SEVEN

Hope for the Future

CHAPTER SIXTEEN

Looking Ahead

So after I've given you all this information on symptoms, treatments, therapies, and complications, you're probably thinking, "Now what? I still have it, right?"

For the moment, yes. After all the treatments and therapies, you may well still have HPV, even if it's undetectable or latent. It's also very possible that you have completely cleared it—we just don't know for sure. We do know that at the moment, no surgical approaches or medicines can cure HPV.

Don't despair, though—help may be on the way. One way in which we're trying is through the use of different kinds of vaccines against HPV. HPV is a tough virus to try to prevent by using a vaccine. There are dozens of HPV types, each affecting different people in different ways. But we're trying.

Before we begin to talk about vaccines, a few words about the immune system are in order. There are two major arms of the immune system: *humoral* and *cell-mediated*. The humoral immune system fights off organisms using antibodies made by your B lymphocytes. If an organism enters your body, your humoral immune system will recognize the organism's proteins as foreign, and the B lymphocytes react by making antibodies. In many cases, these antibodies can attach to the proteins and organisms, blocking the organisms from entering the cells that they're trying to infect. The antibodies are secreted into the blood by the B lymphocytes and are available throughout the body to fight off the organisms. Some B lymphocytes reside in the anogenital tract and secrete antibodies into the cervicovaginal fluids or anal canal to fight organisms directly in those locations.

The cell-mediated arm of the immune system takes a different approach. Instead of sending an antibody to intercept the organism, the body sends cells called T lymphocytes to do the dirty work directly. This typically happens *after* an organism, such as a virus, infects a cell. After the organism enters a cell, the cell exports some of the proteins of the organism to the cell surface. There, the T lymphocytes recognize it as foreign, and the T lymphocytes kill the infected cells through a variety of nasty mechanisms. We've already talked about T lymphocytes in the context of HIV infection, as you may recall. For cell-mediated immunity to happen, then, the T lymphocytes must travel directly to the site of the infection.

Now to the vaccines: In general, there are two different kinds of vaccines: *prophylactic* (also known as preventive) and *therapeutic*. Prophylactic vaccines prevent initial infection by an organism, while therapeutic vaccines are used as treatments of already-existing dysplasia. Most therapeutic vaccines are designed to take advantage of the cell-mediated immune system. Since the organism has already entered the cell, the vaccine can't prevent initial infection, but it can treat already-existing infection and disease due to that infection.

Most prophylactic vaccines are designed to take advantage of the humoral immune system. If the presence of antibodies prevents an organism from entering cells, they can't establish an infection or cause disease. The most familiar vaccinations are prophylactic: Your physician injects a solution containing a small amount of the virus or bacterium. Typically, the virus or bacterium is altered or killed so it doesn't cause active disease. The goal is to stimulate antibodies that will be ready and able to fight off the organism when your body encounters it for real. Another approach is to just inject a piece of the virus or bacterium that is known to stimulate an immune response. Examples of prophylactic or preventive vaccines include those used to prevent measles or hepatitis B infection. When your body comes in contact with the virus—you spend time in close contact with a classmate with measles—your body recognizes the organism and blocks infection with the antibodies stimulated by the vaccine.

What Would a Role Be for a Prophylactic Vaccine for HPV and How Would It Work?

This idea is thrilling in the HPV field. The idea is simple on paper: Take one or more HPV proteins and inject them into young people before they become sexually active, and therefore *before* they have the chance to acquire HPV infection. We've already shown a lot of progress in this work. Several organizations and companies have found that if you make the HPV L1 protein—the most abundant protein in the viral capsid—in the test tube, it assembles itself into a three-dimensional structure that closely resembles the structure of a real mature HPV viral capsid. (You may need to return to chapter 1 to read about viral capsids.)

If you inject these artificial capsids (called *viruslike particles*) they'll stimulate the formation of antibodies that seem to block real HPV viral particles from entering epithelial cells, which is great! And, of course, since the viruslike particles don't contain any HPV DNA, they can't cause an infection themselves.

Several large studies of viruslike particles are in progress. At this point, the data show that they're very safe, but we still don't know how effectively they'll prevent HPV infection. If they work, it would be a tremendous step forward; preventing an infection is much better than treating the disease caused by the infection later on.

Because HPV is spread only by humans, we could eradicate HPV altogether, similar to the eradication of smallpox. Theoretically, if every human was vaccinated against every HPV type, there wouldn't be anyone left to spread it, and it would die out. This is fantasy, of course, for a number of reasons: (1) The vaccine would need to prevent almost all infections; preventing, say, 50 percent of them probably wouldn't be good enough. (2) The viruslike particles are very specific to a given type. To prevent infection with HPV 16, you'd need to vaccinate with a viruslike particle made from the HPV 16 L1 protein. But this might not protect you against HPV 6 or 11. So you'd probably need to be vaccinated with a large cocktail of viruslike particles representing different HPV types. And (3) even if the vaccine works well, it's not certain that it would be used—we don't know at what age we'd need to start vaccinating, and some parents may be reluctant to have their children vaccinated against what is essentially a sexually transmitted agent (Schiller 2000). There are many, many issues here, but this gives you a flavor of what scientists in the HPV field, and their colleagues in the community, will be thinking about over the next few years.

What Would a Role Be for a Therapeutic Vaccine for HPV and How Would It Work?

What about a therapeutic vaccine against HPV? Given all that you now know about the various nasty things that have to be done to treat HPV-associated lesions, wouldn't it be nice if they could be treated with a few vaccine injections instead? This concept, while appealing, is even more challenging than a preventive vaccine. Nevertheless, several organizations and companies are actively testing therapeutic vaccines.

The idea is different here. While the prophylactic vaccines typically use the viruslike particles made from the HPV L1 protein, many therapeutic vaccines use the HPV E7 protein. The E7 protein is continuously made in HPV-infected cells, and pieces of the E7 protein are transported to the cell surface, where they can be recognized by the

T lymphocytes. The therapeutic approach is to inject a person either with the E7 protein or with DNA that will ultimately lead to the production of pieces of the E7 protein by specialized immune helper cells in the body. This will stimulate the proliferation of T lymphocytes primed to recognize and kill the HPV-infected epithelial cells with pieces of E7 on their surface.

This approach has the advantage of being able to kill HPV-infected cells wherever they are in the body—a big plus when you consider that HPV-related lesions can be found in multiple locations at the same time. It also has the advantage of being relatively HPV-specific. In other words, the primed T lymphocytes should only kill the HPV-infected cells and shouldn't harm the uninfected cells.

So far the therapeutic vaccine approach has been shown to be safe. As with the prophylactic vaccines, studies are now determining how well they work. If they work well, technically, you may still carry HPV, but it would remain latent; you'd never get dysplasia or genital warts. The other good news is that patients currently infected with HPV, as well as the uninfected population, could benefit, since HPV-infected people would presumably become less infectious to others.

Like the prophylactic vaccines, these therapeutic vaccines may also be type-specific. If they *do* work, I imagine that someday a sample of the lesional tissue will be removed for HPV testing, and once the HPV type causing the lesion is identified, you'd have your therapeutic vaccine customized to your specific needs. This approach could be useful for dysplasia and for warts. It's even tempting to think it might be useful for patients with invasive cancer.

Researchers constantly test vaccines, and one could be available as early as ten years from now. At this point, they're focused mainly on the most common oncogenic HPVs, 16 and 18, and the genital-wart–causing types, 6 and 11. As the public becomes more aware of the virus and its implications, publicity could increase funding and speed up results for vaccination studies. We can only hope.

What About Antiviral Medicines for HPV?

The development of antiviral therapy has been encouraging as well. Although antiviral drugs won't eradicate HPV, they can slow the replication process, which in turn may prevent the spread and extent of active infection. Again, research is still in the early stages (Phelps et al. 1998).

An example of an interesting compound is indole-3 carbinol—that compound found in broccoli. Early studies documented its use against RRP and moderate dysplasia. More studies are under way, including studies of genital warts. Some studies have reported modest success with vitamin A, retinoic acid, and folic acid. As we said earlier, the role for these dietary supplements in the treatment of HPV-related disease in an otherwise healthy woman is not clear.

Other studies are planned to look at the effect of currently used medications in new ways. For example, imiquimod, which is used for treatment of genital warts, is being tried for the treatment of dysplasia. Even spermicides have been raised as a possible therapeutic approach; some evidence suggests that one of the more commonly used ones—nonoxynol-9—may have some ability to destroy HPV.

Conclusion

As it stands, I hope to see a vaccine within the next ten years. In the meantime, better procedures and medications will continue coming along. With the development of better surgical techniques, new topical medications, and better screening procedures, your general and sexual health will only get better from here. So for now, it's best to focus on behaviors that will reduce your risk of acquiring HPV. If you've already got it, get checked regularly with Paps and do what you can to avoid spreading it to others.

GLOSSARY

Abdominoperineal resection: The removal of the anus and rectum.

Acetowhitening: The process by which HPV-infected tissues turn white in the presence of acetic acid (vinegar).

Adenocarcinoma: A cancer consisting of tumor cells from the glandular epithelium. Examples include endometrial cancer (cancer of the uterus) and cervical adenocarcinoma (cancer of the mucus-producing cells lining the endocervical canal).

AIDS: Acquired immune deficiency syndrome. A syndrome caused by the human immunodeficiency virus in which the body's immunity breaks down.

AIN: Anal intraepithelial neoplasia. A tissue diagnosis in which abnormal squamous cells in the anus are found, which in time may progress to invasive cancer in a small percentage of patients. Another term for this is *anal dysplasia*.

Amniotic fluid: The fluid surrounding a fetus inside the womb.

Anal cancer: Cancer of the epithelium lining the anal canal or the perianal region.

Anoscopy: Procedure in which a colposcope is used to examine the inside of the anus.

Anus: The end opening of the digestive tract.

ASCUS: Atypical squamous cells of undetermined significance. A mildly abnormal Pap smear that may or may not indicate a significant problem.

ASIL: Anal squamous intraepithelial lesions. Abnormal squamous cells in the anus as found in an anal Pap smear.

Basal cells: The cells located in the bottom, or lowest layer, of the epithelium.

Benign: A condition that will not lead to the development of cancer.

Bethesda system: The system currently used by pathologists to rate the levels of an abnormal Pap smear.

Bilateral oophorectomy: The surgical removal of both ovaries.

Biological therapy: Therapy in which vitamins and drugs are administered to boost the body's natural defenses.

Biopsy: A sample of tissue. Also describes the act of removing a sample of tissue.

Bowenoid papulosis of the penis: Small areas of severe penile dysplasia that may progress to invasive cancer in a small percentage of patients.

Cancer: General term for the unrestrained growth of abnormal, malignant cells in the body's tissues.

Capsid: The protein shell covering a virus.

Carbon dioxide laser: A laser often used to ablate genital warts or treat dysplasia.

Carcinogen: Any substance, such as nicotine, known to contribute to the formation of cancerous cells.

Carcinoma in situ: Also known as Stage 0 cancer or "cancer in waiting." These are not truly cancerous, but may progress to invasive cancer over time if left untreated.

Cell: Smallest unit of living organisms capable of independent function.

Cervical cancer: Cancer of the epithelium lining the cervix or endocervical canal.

Cervical incompetence: A weakened cervix that may be incapable of holding a fetus, inducing miscarriage.

Cervical intraepithelial neoplasia (CIN): A tissue diagnosis in which abnormal squamous cells in the cervix are found, which in time may progress to invasive cancer in a small percentage of patients. Also called *cervical dysplasia.*

Cervical portio: A part of the cervix; for example, the *portio vaginalis* is the part of the cervix contained within the vagina.

Cervical stenosis: Constriction of the cervical opening, causing uterine pain and impairing menstrual blood flow; usually results from injury to the tissues.

Cervix: The "neck," or opening, of the uterus.

Cesarean section: The surgical delivery of a baby, performed by cutting through the abdominal wall.

Chemotherapy: The use of chemicals or drugs to kill cancerous cells.

Chronic: Describes a condition of long duration.

Cisplatin: A drug commonly used in chemotherapy for cervical cancer.

Clinical infection: An active, visible infection; the most infectious expression of a virus.

Clinical trial: A series of experimental, unproven therapies for the treatment or comfort of patients.

Clitoris: A protuberance in the vulva which is considered to be the "female penis" and a source of sexual stimulation.

Colostomy: The surgical creation of an opening in the abdomen to allow the evacuation of intestinal wastes (in the absence of a rectum or anus).

Colposcope: A microscope with a built-in light used for examining the vagina, cervix, and vulva.

Colposcopy: The procedure using a colposcope to examine the vagina, cervix, and vulva for suspicious lesions, usually accompanied by a biopsy of cervical tissue.

Columnar cells: The mucus-producing cells lining the endocervical canal and in the basal layer of the transformation zone.

Condyloma acuminata: Genital warts, often caused by HPV types 6 and 11.

Conization: The excision of a conical portion of cervical tissue for curative and/or diagnostic purposes.

Cryotherapy/cryosurgery: The procedure of freezing tissue to kill and remove abnormal tissues or growths.

CSIL: Same as cervical dysplasia, but refers to the abnormal cells found on a cervical Pap smear.

Curettage: The removal of tissue with a spoon-shaped instrument, usually to remove abnormal tissue or obtain a biopsy.

Curette: The spoon-shaped instrument used to scrape cell samples from the inner wall of body cavities.

Cutaneous warts: Warts that grow on the skin.

D&C: Dilatation and curettage. Procedure in which the cervix is dilated so a curette may scrape the uterine lining.

DNA virus: Virus in which the nucleic acid is made up of DNA. Includes HPV and herpes simplex virus.

Dysplasia: An area of abnormal intraepithelial cells, indicating an active HPV infection in the genitals. Another term for this is *intraepithelial neoplasia.*

Electrodessication: Procedure in which an electrical current destroys a wart.

Endocervical curettage: Scraping of the inside lining of the endocervical canal with a sharp curette.

Endophytic warts: Warts that grow into the skin, such as plantar warts.

Epidemiology: A branch of medicine that deals with the development, distribution, and control of disease in a population.

Episome: When the genome of a virus or other DNA remains separate from the human genome DNA.

Epitheliotropic: Having a special affinity for epithelial cells.

Epithelium: The closely packed layer of skin cells covering the external surface and the lining of several internal organs.

Etiology: The cause of something.

Exophytic warts: Warts that grow out of the skin.

External radiation therapy: Cancer treatment in which radiation is directed at the affected area of the patient's body.

Genome: The sum total of all of the genes of an organism.

HIV: Human immunodeficiency virus. The virus that causes AIDS.

Hormone replacement therapy: The administration of hormones to balance a woman's body chemistry during or after menopause or a menopause-inducing condition (such as hysterectomy).

HSIL: High-grade squamous intraepithelial lesions. A diagnosis of moderately or severely abnormal cells on a Pap smear, often indicates the presence of a lesion that could progress to invasive cancer if left untreated.

HSV: Herpes simplex virus. A virus that causes sores in the genitalia, mouth, or other mucous membranes.

Hybrid Capture II: The commercially available test that distinguishes oncogenic from nononcogenic HPV types.

Hysterectomy: The removal of the uterus. **Radical:** Removal of the uterus, cervix, upper third of the vagina, fallopian tubes, ovaries, and all pelvic lymph nodes through an abdominal incision. **Total:** Removal of the uterus and cervix only through an abdominal incision. **Vaginal:** Removal of the uterus through the vagina.

Imiquimod: A topical genital wart medication designed to stimulate local immunity and thus reduce the size and frequency of genital warts. Trade name is Aldara.

Interferon: A naturally occurring molecule that has antiviral activity.

Internal radiation therapy: Cancer therapy in which a radioactive substance is placed within the cancerous tissue. Also known as *intracavitary* or *interstitial radiation therapy*.

Interstitial radiation therapy: See *internal radiation therapy*.

Intracavitary radiation therapy: See *internal radiation therapy.*

Intraepithelial: Within the epithelium or skin layer. Remains above the basement membrane and is not cancerous.

Intraepithelial neoplasia: An area of abnormal intraepithelial cells, often indicates an active HPV infection in the genitals. Also called *dysplasia.*

Invasive cancer: Condition in which cancerous cells have invaded the basement membrane and invaded underlying tissues.

Irradiation: Use of radioactive energy to kill cancer cells.

Keratinized, keratotic: Rough feel or appearance due to the presence of a hard coating produced by the epithelial cells known as keratin.

Labia majora: The two outer lips protecting the inner vulva.

Labia minora: The two inner lips of the vulva protecting the clitoris and vestibule.

Larynx: The voice box.

Latent infection: A condition in which the virus is present but there are no signs of active infection. The patient is probably not infectious. Another word for latent is *dormant.*

LEEP: Loop electrocautery excision procedure. The excision of abnormal tissue by using an electrical loop.

Lesion: General term for any abnormal change in the structure of tissues due to disease.

LSIL: Low-grade squamous intraepithelial lesions. A diagnosis of mildly abnormal cells on a Pap smear.

Lymph node dissection: The removal of lymph nodes in the pelvis for diagnosis and sometimes to help prevent cancer spread.

Malignant: Another word for cancerous.

Menopause: The permanent cessation of menstruation.

Metaplasia: Replacement of cells of one type by cells of another type, such as replacement of columnar cells by squamous cells.

Metastasis: The process by which cancerous tumors spread to tissues distant from the original cancer.

Metastasize: To spread by metastasis, by the bloodstream or through the lymph nodes.

Mons pubis: The layer of fatty tissue over the pubic area.

Mucosal: Being of a mucous membrane, such as the moist skin surfaces of the mouth, vagina, or anus.

Neoplasia: The abnormal cell growth resulting in a tumor.

Nucleus: The control center or "brain" of a cell.

Oncogenic: Capable of contributing to the development of cancer.

Palliative therapy: Therapy designed to treat symptoms and make a patient more comfortable, rather than cure the illness.

Pap smear: The smear of cervical, vaginal, or anal cells.

Pap test: The examination of cells scraped from the cervical, vaginal, and anal walls.

Papillae: Fingerlike projections.

Papilloma: A benign tumor growing from the epithelium of skin and mucous membranes, usually associated with HPV.

Papule: A small, solid elevation of skin that can grow from superficial or deep layers of skin.

Pelvic examination: The procedure in which a physician examines the vulva, vagina, cervix, ovaries, and uterus.

Pelvic exenteration: The surgical removal of the vagina, cervix, uterus, ovaries, lower colon, and rectum.

Penile cancer: The development of cancerous cells in the penis.

Perianal: Describing the area surrounding the opening of the anal canal.

Perinatal transmission: The transmission of a disease from mother to infant during childbirth.

Perineum: The area between the vulva (female) or scrotum (male) and anus.

Podofilox: A patient-applied therapy for genital warts that works by slowing down cell division. Also known as podophyllotoxin. Trade name is Condylox.

Podophyllin: A provider-administered therapy for genital warts, contains podophyllotoxin.

Prepuce: The fold of skin overlapping the clitoris (female) or penis (male). Also called the foreskin.

Prevention trials: Clinical trials to test vaccines and other preventive drugs.

Punch biopsy: The procedure in which a sharp, round "punch" instrument removes a sample of skin for testing.

Quality-of-life trials: Clinical trials to test palliative therapies.

Radiation therapy: The use of radioactive rays or material to kill abnormal cells.

Radical vulvectomy: The removal of the entire vulva, including the labia majora and minora, clitoris, and perineum.

Rectum: The area between the lower colon and the anus.

Recurrent: A condition that returns after treatment.

Recurrent respiratory papillomatosis: The persistent growth of benign tumors in the respiratory tract.

Reinfection: The reintroduction of a virus.

Screening trials: Clinical trials to test new screening methods.

Scrotum: The sac of skin enclosing the testicles.

Shaft: The midsection of the penis.

Skinning vulvectomy: The removal of the top layer of vulvar skin to preserve functional and cosmetic results.

Squamous: Flat, or scalelike, cells of the skin or epithelium.

Squamous cell carcinoma: Abnormal, malignant transformation of squamous cells of the skin or epithelium.

Staging: The process used to determine how advanced a cancer is.

Stroma: The cells and connective tissues underneath skin layer.

Supportive care trials: See *quality-of-life trials*.

Terminal: Fatal.

Trachea: The tube extending from the larynx to the bronchi; also called the windpipe.

Trachelectomy: The surgical removal of the cervix.

Transformation zone: The area in which round columnar cells transform into the flatter squamous cells. The most common area of HPV infection, cervical or anal dysplasia, and cancer.

Transmission: The act of passing an infectious agent from one host to another.

Treatment trials: Clinical trials to test new treatment methods.

Trichloroacetic acid (TCA): A provider-administered therapy for genital warts and other HPV-associated lesions.

Tumor: An overgrowth of abnormal cells.

Urethra: The canal carrying urine from the bladder to the outside of the body.

Urethral meatus: The opening of the urethra.

Uterus: The organ used for carrying a fetus.

Vagina: The sheathlike organ between the cervix and vulva; also called the birth canal.

Vaginal birth: To give birth through the vagina.

Vaginal cancer: The development of cancerous cells in the vagina.

Vaginectomy: The surgical removal of the vagina.

VAIN: Vaginal intraepithelial neoplasia. A tissue diagnosis in which abnormal squamous cells in the vagina are found, which in time may progress to invasive cancer in a small percentage of patients. Also called vaginal dysplasia.

Vestibule: The space between the labia minora; the opening of the vagina and urethra.

VIN: Vulvar intraepithelial neoplasia. A tissue diagnosis in which abnormal squamous cells in the vulva are found, which in time may progress to invasive cancer in a small percentage of patients. Also called vulvar dysplasia.

Virus: An infectious agent consisting of a genome and protein coating that thrives and replicates only in living cells.

Vulva: The outer female genitalia, including the mons pubis, labia majora and minora, prepuce, clitoris, and vestibule.

Vulvar cancer: The development of cancerous cells in the vulva.

Vulvectomy: The surgical removal of all or part of the vulva.

Warts: Benign growth from the epithelium of mucous membranes or skin; caused by HPV.

Wide local excision: The surgical removal of diseased tissue and some surrounding normal tissue.

APPENDIX A

Choosing Your Gynecologist

When choosing your gynecologist, don't just pick a name out of your insurance carrier's book. If you've been living in a place for a long time, my first advice would be to ask women you trust for referrals. Depending on your relationship with the woman, she'll probably be more than willing to give you details on her doctor's personality. If you already have a primary-care physician you trust, ask him or her for referrals; if you're new to an area, you can call 1-800-DOCTORS to get referrals, and the web is a great place for research. Go to *www.1800doctors.com*.

You are entitled to an interview with your gynecologist, an introduction in which you can feel him or her out and decide if you're mutually compatible. If after your first exam you have any misgivings about your doctor, find a new one. An atmosphere of mistrust and caution on the table doesn't do either one of you any good.

"During my first visit with one doctor, she couldn't really meet my eyes," says Beth, age twenty-four. "She seemed a little nervous about talking with me about sex, which I thought was kind of weird. But I kept going to her anyway, and when my Pap smear came out abnormal, she didn't give me any information—just threw some pamphlets at me and said not to worry about it. The next doctor I picked was a woman who a friend recommended to me, and she's been great."

During your first visit with a new gynecologist, it's natural to feel a little apprehensive. After all, a stranger is putting his or her hands in the most intimate part of your body. But a good doctor should make you feel comfortable, relaxed, and open. "I was a little nervous at first, since he was a man, but then he talked to me about college the whole time and loosened me up," says Alice, age twenty-eight.

Your gynecologist should be a trusted authority figure in your life—someone who offers constructive medical advice, not judgments. If she tells you to quit smoking, use contraception, or to consider the risks of having multiple sexual partners, she's giving you constructive medical advice. Judgmental attitudes, however, don't belong in the doctor's office.

When you find the right doctor, you'll develop an atmosphere of trust that probably doesn't exist with anyone else in your life. Before going into your exam, make a list of concerns and questions you'd like to address, no matter how silly you think they may be. Even if that little itch turns out to be nothing, you'll at least feel better for knowing.

APPENDIX B

Pelvic Self-Examination

Although you may feel strange at first, working a pelvic self-examination into your monthly health routine—along with a breast exam—can alert you and your doctor to infections like HPV or HSV as well as early cancerous changes. If you find that doing the exam yourself is too difficult or awkward, your partner may be able to help you.

The best time to do a self-exam is in the middle of your menstrual cycle; you should make a point of doing it at the same time every month, since alterations in your hormones can affect the amount of discharge and the color of your vagina and cervix.

Remember that the self-examination does *not* replace an annual pelvic exam by a doctor.

You'll need:

- A hand mirror
- A strong light

- A vaginal lubricant
- A plastic speculum (you can buy one at a pharmacy that sells medical supplies)
- An antiseptic soap or alcohol

Vulvar Exam

The vulvar exam is fairly simple to perform, requiring only the light and a mirror.

1. Find a place to relax. If you feel uncomfortable performing an exam with anyone around, wait until you're alone in your apartment or house; tension can affect the exam.
2. Place the mirror at your feet.
3. Shining the light into the mirror so it illuminates your pelvis, examine your vulva for any irregularities. Look for discolorations, bumps, growths, or irritations. Use your hand to feel the texture of the area; some bumps are a part of your natural form, so it may take a few examinations to know which ones are normal and which are unusual.
4. If you notice any irregularities, talk to your doctor about it.

Vaginal and Cervical Exam

After performing a vulvar exam, you can move on to the vaginal and cervical exam, which is more difficult. **Note that these examinations should not replace your regular follow-up with your doctor.**

1. Lie back.
2. Bend your knees, with your feet wide apart.
3. Lubricate the speculum, and insert it into your vagina in the closed position. Experiment to find the most comfortable position for inserting the speculum.
4. Once the speculum is inserted, grab the shorter section of the handle and firmly pull it toward you until it opens inside your vagina.
5. Push down on the outside section until you hear a click, while keeping a firm hold on the speculum. The speculum is now locked in place.
6. Place the mirror at your feet so that you can see your vagina. Move the speculum, while shining the flashlight into the mirror, until you can see your cervix and vaginal walls in the mirror.
7. Take note of the color of your cervix, as well as any vaginal secretions.
8. After your examination is complete, remove the speculum, either in the closed or open position, whichever is most comfortable for you.
9. Thoroughly wash the speculum with antiseptic soap or alcohol and store for your next self-exam.

APPENDIX C

Penile Self-Examination

Although only a doctor can conduct a thorough penile examination, a man can do regular self-examinations. I recommend this especially if you know you've been exposed to HPV. Regular self-examinations make you aware of the natural bumps and ridges on your body and can alert you to any unusual changes. You may find it helpful for your partner to also examine the area.

Keep in mind, though, that you and your partner can identify the obvious lesions, but smaller warts and subclinical lesions do require a doctor's expertise.

You'll need:

- A hand mirror
- A strong light
- A magnifying glass, if available

Penile Self-Exam

1. Wash the area thoroughly, including the pubic hair and perineum, and dry off.
2. Using your hand, feel for any unusual bumps or ridges on the shaft, head, and underside of your penis. If you have a foreskin, feel along its inside and outside. Feel through the pubic area and perineum, as well, for any unusual bumps or growths.
3. You might want to perform a testicle examination at this time, as well; gently roll each testicle between your thumb and fingers, feeling for any lumps or enlargements.
4. Direct bright light at your genitalia. Thoroughly examine the surface of your penis and surrounding areas for reddish or darker areas; bumps that may look like pimples; open sores; or warts.
5. Spread the pubic hair and thoroughly examine the area for any of these symptoms.
6. Using a mirror, examine the underside of your penis and perineum, the area between your scrotum and anus.
7. If you see any unusual growths, dark or reddish areas, open sores, or warts, notify your doctor immediately.

APPENDIX D

Resources

Below is a list of solid resources for information on Pap smears, cervical disease, HPV, genital warts, clinical trials, and support groups. This is by no means all-inclusive, so talk to your doctor about other resources!

About.com
www.womenshealth.about.com

AfraidToAsks's Sexually Transmitted Disease Guide
www.afraidtoask.com/std.htm

Alternatives in Gynecology
15195 National Avenue, Suite 201
Los Gatos, CA 95032
408-358-2788
www.gynalternatives.com

American Medical Association
Sexually Transmitted Disease Information Center
515 North State Street
Chicago, IL 60610
312-464-5000
www.ama-assn.org/special/std/std.htm

American Social Health Association
National HPV and Cervical Cancer Prevention
  Resource Center
P.O. Box 13827
Research Triangle Park, NC 27709
Hotline: 1-877-HPV-5868
www.ashastd.org or *www.iwannaknow.org* (for teens)

American Society of Clinical Pathologists
2100 West Harrison Street
Chicago, IL 60612
312-738-1336
www.ascp.org

Centers for Disease Control
www.cdc.gov/nchstp/dstd/disease_info.htm#hpv

iVillage and AllHealth
www.allhealth.com

Thrive
www.thrive.com

Woman's Diagnostic Cyber Network
www.wdxcyber.com

CANCER RESOURCES

National Cancer Institute
Public Inquiries Office
Building 31, Room 10A03
31 Center Drive, MSC 2580
Bethesda, MD 20892-2580
Hotline: 1-800-4-CANCER
www.cancer.gov

National Cervical Cancer Coalition (NCCC)
16501 Sherman Way, Suite 110
Van Nuys, CA 91406
Hotline: 1-800-685-5531
www.nccc-online.org

ONLINE SUPPORT GROUPS

AllHealth
www.boards.allhealth.com

Thrive
www.boards.thriveonline.com

Yahoo
www.clubs.yahoo.com/clubs/hpv
www.clubs.yahoo.com/clubs/hpvclinicaltrialsandtestsinfo

REFERENCES

Allen, D. G., R. S. Planner, P. T. Tang, J. P. Scurry, and T. Weerasiri. 1995. "Invasive cervical cancer in pregnancy." *Australian and New Zealand Journal of Obstetrics and Gynecology* 35, no. 4 (November): 408–12.

American Social Health Association. 1999. "Consumer/patient fact sheet." National HPV and Cervical Cancer Prevention Resource Center, Research Triangle Park, North Carolina.

Apgar, B. S. 1996. "Differentiating normal and abnormal findings of the vulva." *American Family Physician* 53, no. 4 (March): 1171–80.

Barrasso, R. 2000. "Colposcopic terminology: Which and why." Paper presented at the 18th International Papillomavirus Conference and HPV Clinical Workshop jointly with the 12th Meeting of the AEPCC, Barcelona, Spain, July.

Basta, A., K. Adamek, and K. Pitynski. 1999. "Intraepithelial neoplasia and early stage vulvar cancer: Epidemiological, clinical and virological observations." *European Journal of Gynecological Oncology* 20, no. 2: 111–14.

Bosanquet, N., D. V. Coleman, C. J. Dore, G. Douglass, and L. J. Magee. 1999. "Assessment of automated primary screening on

PAPNET of cervical smears in the PRISMATIC trial." *The Lancet* 353, no. 9162 (April): 1381–85.

Boxman, I. L., A. Hogewonig, L. H. Mulder, J. N. Bouwes Bavinck, and J. ter Schegget. 1999. "Detection of human papillomavirus types 6 and 11 in pubic and perianal hair from patients with genital warts." *Journal of Clinical Microbiology* 37, no. 7 (July): 2270–73.

Campion, M. J., M. D. Greenberg, and T.I.G. Kazamel. 1996. Clinical manifestations and natural history of genital human papillomavirus infections. *Obstetrics and Gynecology Clinics of North America* 23: 783.

Cason, J., J. N. Kaye, R. J. Jewers, P. K. Jambo, J. M. Bible, B. Kell, B. Shergill, F. Pakarian, K. S. Raju, and J. M. Best. 1995. "Perinatal infection and persistence of human papillomavirus types 16 and 18 in infants." *Journal of Medical Virology* 47, no. 3 (November): 209–18.

Connor, J. P. 1998. "Noninvasive cervical cancer complicating pregnancy." *Obstetrics and Gynecology Clinics of North America* 25, no. 2 (June): 331–42.

Covens, A., P. Shaw, J. Murphy, D. DePetrillo, G. Lickrish, S. Laframboise, and B. Rosen. 1999. "Is radical trachelectomy a safe alternative to radical hysterectomy for patients with stage IA-B carcinoma of the cervix?" *Cancer* 86, no. 11 (December): 2273–79.

Cox, J. T. 1998. "New developments in cervical cancer screening and prevention." *Journal of the National Cancer Institute* 90, no. 23 (December): 1839–40.

Dargent, D., X. Martin, A. Sacchetoni, and P. Mathevet. 2000. "Laparoscopic vaginal radical trachelectomy: A treatment to preserve the fertility of cervical carcinoma patients." *Cancer* 88, no. 8 (April): 1877–82.

Denny, L., L. Kuhn, A. Pollack, and T. C. Wright. 2000. "HPV DNA testing as a primary screening test in low resource settings." Paper presented at the 18th International Papillomavirus Conference and HPV Clinical Workshop jointly with the 12th Meeting of the AEPCC, Barcelona, Spain, July.

De Palo, G. 2000. "Colposcopy in the vulvo-vaginal HPV infection." Paper presented at the 18th International Papillomavirus Conference and HPV Clinical Workshop jointly with the 12th Meeting of the AEPCC, Barcelona, Spain, July.

Diakomanolis, E. 2000. "Treatment of VAIN." Paper presented at the 18th International Papillomavirus Conference and HPV Clinical Workshop jointly with the 12th Meeting of the AEPCC, Barcelona, Spain, July.

Dox, Ida G., June L. Melloni, and Harrison H. Sheld. 2000. *Melloni's illustrated dictionary of obstetrics and gynecology.* Pearl River, N.Y.: Parthenon Publishing.

Edwards, C. L., G. Tortolero-Luna, A. C. Linares, A. Malpica, V. Baker, E. Cook, E. Johnson, and M. Follen Mitchell. 1996. "Vulvar intraepithelial neoplasia and vulvar cancer." *Obstetrics and Gynecology Clinics of North America* 23, no. 2 (June): 295–324.

El-Bastawissi, A. Y., T. M. Becker, and J. R. Daling, 1999. "Effect of cervical carcinoma in situ and its management on pregnancy outcome." *Obstetrics and Gynecology* 93: 207–12.

Ferenczy, A., and A. B. Johnson. 1996. "Tissue effects and host response." *Obstetrics and Gynecology Clinics of North America* 23, no. 4 (December): 759–82.

Franco, E. L. 1999. "Epidemiology and natural history of HPV-induced disease." Paper presented at the 17th International Papillomavirus Conference, Charleston, South Carolina, January.

———. 1996. "Epidemiology of anogenital warts and cancer."

Obstetrics and Gynecology Clinics of North America 23, no. 3 (September): 597–624.

Ghaly, A.F.F., I. D. Duncan, and S. M. Nicoll. 1999. "Should women with genital condyloma acuminata have routine diagnostic colposcopy in addition to cervical smear screening?" *Journal of Obstetrics and Gynecology* 19, no. 5 (September): 500–502.

Gissman, L. 2000. "Vaccination against HPV: Evidence and prospects." Paper presented at the 18th International Papillomavirus Conference and HPV Clinical Workshop jointly with the 12th Meeting of the AEPCC, Barcelona, Spain, July.

Giuliano, A. R., and S. Gapstur. 1998. "Can cervical dysplasia and cancer be prevented with nutrients?" *Nutrition Reviews* 56, no. 1 (January): 9–16.

Goldie, S. J., K. M. Kuntz, M. C. Weinstein, K. A. Freedberg, and J. M. Palefsky. 2000. "The clinical benefits and cost-effectiveness of screening for anal squamous intraepithelial lesions and anal squamous cell cancer in homosexual and bisexual men." *American Journal of Medicine*, 108:634–41.

Goldie, S. J., K. M. Kuntz, M. C. Weinstein, K. A. Freedberg, M. L. Welton, and J. M. Palefsky. 1999. "The clinical-effectiveness and cost-effectiveness of screening for anal squamous intraepithelial lesions in homosexual and bisexual HIV-positive men." *JAMA* 281:1822–29.

Greene, P., D. Smith, P. Kratt, and K. Donovan. 2000. "Behavioral issues in cervical cancer prevention." Paper presented at the 18th International Papillomavirus Conference and HPV Clinical Workshop jointly with the 12th Meeting of the AEPCC, Barcelona, Spain, July.

Groopman, J. 1999. "Contagion: A sometimes lethal epidemic that condoms can't stop." *The New Yorker* (September): 34–49.

Herrero, R. 2000. "HPV and cancer of the lower genital tract."

Paper presented at the 18th International Papillomavirus Conference and HPV Clinical Workshop jointly with the 12th Meeting of the AEPCC, Barcelona, Spain, July.

————. 2000. "HPV and cancer of the upper aerodigestive tract." Paper presented at the 18th International Papillomavirus Conference and HPV Clinical Workshop jointly with the 12th Meeting of the AEPCC, Barcelona, Spain, July.

Hildesheim, A., C. L. Han, L. A. Brinton, R. J. Kurman, and J. T. Schiller. 1997. "Human papillomavirus type 16 and risk of preinvasive and invasive vulvar cancer: Results from a sero-epidemiological case-control study." *Obstetrics and Gynecology* 90, no. 5 (November): 748–54.

Jay, N., J. M. Berry, C. J. Hogeboom, E. A. Holly, T. M. Darragh, and J. M. Palefsky. 1997. "Colposcopic appearance of anal squamous intraepithelial lesions: Relationship to histopathology." *Diseases of the Colon and Rectum* 40, no. 8 (August): 919–28.

Kahn, J. A., and S. J. Emans. 1999. "Pap smears in adolescents: To screen or not to screen?" *Pediatrics* 103, no. 3 (March): 673–74.

Kashima, H. K., P. Mounts, and K. Shah. 1996. "Recurrent respiratory papillomatosis." *Obstetrics and Gynecology Clinics of North America* 23, no. 3 (September): 699–706.

Klencke, B. 2000. "HPV in anal and penile cancers." Paper presented at the 18th International Papillomavirus Conference and HPV Clinical Workshop jointly with the 12th Meeting of the AEPCC, Barcelona, Spain, July.

Kwasniewska, A., A. Tukendorf, and M. Semczuk. 1997. "Frequency of HPV infection and GSH levels in plasma of women with cervical dysplasia." *European Journal of Gynecological Oncology* 18, no. 3: 196–99.

Langley, P. C., S. K. Tyring, and M. H. Smith. 1999. "The cost-effectiveness of patient-applied versus provider-administered intervention strategies for the treatment of external genital warts." *American Journal of Managed Care* 5, no. 1 (January): 69–77.

Lazo, P. A. 2000. "Genetic damage in cervical carcinoma." Paper presented at the 18th International Papillomavirus Conference and HPV Clinical Workshop jointly with the 12th Meeting of the AEPCC, Barcelona, Spain, July.

Lowy, D. R. 2000. "HPV vaccination as a novel preventive strategy." Paper presented at the 18th International Papillomavirus Conference and HPV Clinical Workshop jointly with the 12th Meeting of the AEPCC, Barcelona, Spain, July.

Meirow, D., S. J. Fasouliotis, D. Nugent, J. G. Schenker, R. G. Gosden, and A. J. Rutherford. 1999. "A laparoscopic technique for obtaining ovarian cortical biopsy specimens for fertility conservation in patients with cancer." *Fertility and Sterility* 71, no. 5 (May): 948–51.

Miller, A. B. 2000. "Screening options: Summary of the international review conferences held in 1999." Paper presented at the 18th International Papillomavirus Conference and HPV Clinical Workshop jointly with the 12th meeting of the AEPCC, Barcelona, Spain, July.

Monaghan, J. 1999. "Time to add chemotherapy to radiotherapy for cervical cancer." *The Lancet* 353, no. 9161 (April): 1288–89.

Moscicki, A. B., J. M. Palefsky, J. Gonzales, and G. K. Schoolnik. 1990. "Human papillomavirus infection in sexually active adolescent females: Prevalence and risk factors." *Pediatric Research* 28, no. 5: 507–13.

Nakagawa, K., Y. Aoki, T. Kusama, N. Ban, S. Nakagawa, and Y. Sasaki. 1997. "Radiotherapy during pregnancy: Effects on fetuses and neonates." *Clinical Therapeutics* 19, no. 4 (July–August): 770–77.

Onwudiegwu, U., A. Bako, and A. Oyewumi. 1999. "Cervical cancer: A neglected health tragedy." *Journal of Obstetrics and Gynecology* 19, no. 1 (January): 61–64.

Osorio, M. T. 2000. "Treatment of high-grade SIL." Paper presented at the 18th International Papillomavirus Conference and HPV Clinical Workshop jointly with the 12th Meeting of the AEPCC, Barcelona, Spain, July.

Palefsky, J. M., and R. Barrasso. 1996. "HPV infection and disease in men." *Obstetrics and Gynecology Clinics of North America* 23, no. 4 (December): 895–916.

Palefsky, J. M., E. A. Holly, J. Gonzales, J. Berline, D. K. Ahn, and J. S. Greenspan. 1991. "Detection of human papillomavirus DNA in anal intraepithelial neoplasia and anal cancer." *Cancer Research* 51 (February): 1014–19.

Palefsky, J. M., E. A. Holly, C. J. Hogeboom, M. L. Ralston, M. M. DaCosta, R. Botts, J. M. Berry, N. Jay, and T. M. Darragh. 1998. "Viral, immunologic and clinical parameters in the incidence and progression of anal squamous intraepithelial lesions in HIV-positive and HIV-negative homosexual men." *Journal of Acquired Immune Deficiency Syndrome* 17:314–19.

Palefsky, J. M., E. A. Holly, M. L. Ralston, S. P. Arthur, N. Jay, J. M. Berry, M. M. DaCosta, R. Botts, and T. M. Darragh. 1998. "Anal squamous intraepithelial lesions among HIV-positive and HIV-negative homosexual and bisexual men: Prevalence and risk factors." *Journal of Acquired Immune Deficiency Syndrome* 17:320–26.

Palefsky, J. M., E. A. Holly, M. L. Ralston, M. Da Costa, and R. M. Greenblatt. 2001. "Prevalence and risk factors for anal HPV infection in HIV-positive and high-risk HIV-negative women." *Journal of Infectious Diseases* 183:383–391.

Palefsky, J. M., E. A. Holly, M. L. Ralston, and N. Jay. 1998. "Prevalence and risk factors for human papillomavirus infection of the anal canal in HIV-positive and HIV-negative homosexual men." *Journal of Infectious Diseases* 177:361–67.

Palefsky, J. M., E. A. Holly, M. L. Ralston, N. Jay, J. M. Berry, and T. M. Darragh. 1998. "High incidence of anal high-grade squamous intraepithelial lesions among HIV-positive and HIV-negative homosexual/bisexual men." *AIDS* 12:495–503.

Palefsky, J. M., H. Minkoff, L. A. Kalish, A. Levine, H. S. Sacks, P. Garcia, M. Young, S. Melnick, P. Miotti, and R. Burk. 1999. "Cervicovaginal human papillomavirus infection in HIV-positive and high-risk HIV-negative women." *Journal of the National Cancer Institute* 91:226–35.

Perry, C. M., and H. M. Lamb. 1999. "Topical imiquimod: A review of its use in genital warts." *Drugs* 58, no. 2 (August): 375–90.

Phelps, W. C., J. A. Barnes, and D. C. Lobe. 1998. "Molecular targets for human papillomaviruses: Prospects for antiviral therapy." *Antiviral Chemistry and Chemotherapy* 9: 359–77.

Pinto, A. P., L. B. Signorello, C. P. Crum, B. L. Harlow, F. Abrao, and L. L. Villa. 1999. "Squamous cell carcinoma of the vulva in Brazil: Prognostic importance of host and viral variables." *Gynecologic Oncology* 74, no. 1 (July): 61–67.

Pollack, A. E. 2000. "Dignity vs. disaster: The complex lives of developing country women with cervical cancer." Paper presented at the 18th International Papillomavirus Conference and HPV Clinical Workshop jointly with the 12th Meeting of the AEPCC, Barcelona, Spain, July.

Ponten, J., and Z. Guo. 1998. "Precancer of the human cervix." *Cancer Surveys* 32: 201–29.

Prendiville, W. "LSIL: To treat or not to treat." Paper presented at the 18th International Papillomavirus Conference and HPV Clinical Workshop jointly with the 12th Meeting of the AEPCC, Barcelona, Spain, July.

Reid, R. 1996. "The management of genital condylomas, intraepithelial neoplasia, and vulvodynia." *Obstetrics and Gynecology Clinics of North America* 23, no. 4 (December): 917–91.

Ronnett, B. M., M. M. Manos, J. E. Ransley, B. J. Fetterman, W. K. Kinney, L. B. Hurley, J. S. Ngai, R. J. Kurman, and M. E. Sherman. 1999. "Atypical glandular cells of undetermined significance (AGUS): Cytopathologic features, histopathologic results, and human papillomavirus DNA detection." *Human Pathology* 30, no. 7 (July): 816–26.

Roy, M. and M. Plante. 1998. "Pregnancies after radical vaginal trachelectomy for early-stage cervical cancer." *American Journal of Obstetrics and Gynecology* 179, no. 6 (December): 1491–96.

Sasieni, P. 2000. "A systematic review of the role of HPV testing within a cervical screening program." Paper presented at the 18th International Papillomavirus Conference and HPV Clinical Workshop jointly with the 12th Meeting of the AEPCC, Barcelona, Spain, July.

Saunders, C. S. 2000. "A breakthrough in cervical cancer treatment." *Patient Care* 34, no. 2 (January): 70–90.

Schiller, J. T. 2000. "HPV vaccines in the year 2000 and ahead." Paper presented at the 18th International Papillomavirus Conference and HPV Clinical Workshop jointly with the 12th Meeting of the AEPCC, Barcelona, Spain, July.

Shah, K. V. 1998. "Do human papillomavirus infections cause oral cancer?" *Journal of the National Cancer Institute* 90, no. 21 (November): 1585–86.

———. 2000. "What are human papillomaviruses?" Paper presented at the 18th International Papillomavirus Conference and HPV Clinical Workshop jointly with the 12th Meeting of the AEPCC, Barcelona, Spain, July.

Shrier, L. A. 1998. "Commentary on 'Evaluation of vaginal infections in adolescent women: Can it be done without a speculum?' " *Pediatrics* 102 (October): 939–44.

Singer, A. 2000. "The polarprobe: Emerging technologies for cervical cancer screening." Paper presented at the 18th International Papillomavirus Conference and HPV Clinical Workshop jointly with the 12th meeting of the AEPCC, Barcelona, Spain, July.

Sood, A. K., and J. I. Sorosky. 1998. "Invasive cervical cancer complicating pregnancy: How to manage the dilemma." *Obstetrics and Gynecology Clinics of North America* 25, no. 2 (June): 343–52.

Sood, A. K., J. I. Sorosky, S. Krogman, B. Anderson, J. Benda, and R. E. Buller. 1996. "Surgical management of cervical cancer complicating pregnancy: A case-control study." *Gynecologic Oncology* 63, no. 3 (December): 294–98.

Sood, A.K., J. I. Sorosky, N. Mayr, B. Anderson, R. E. Buller, and J. Niebyl. 2000. "Cervical cancer diagnosed shortly after pregnancy: Prognostic variables and delivery routes." *Obstetrics and Gynecology* 95, no. 6 (June): 832–38.

Tenti, P., R. Zappatore, P. Migliora, A. Spinillo, C. Belloni, and L. Carneval. 1999. "Perinatal transmission of human papillomavirus from gravidas with latent infections." *Obstetrics & Gynecology* 93:475–9.

Trimble, C. L., A. Hildesheim, L. A. Brinton, K. V. Shah, and R. J. Kurman. 1996. "Heterogeneous etiology of squamous carcinoma of the vulva." *Obstetrics and Gynecology* 87, no. 1 (January): 59–64.

Tseng, C. J., C. C. Liang, Y. K. Soong, and C. C. Pao. 1998. "Perinatal transmission of human papillomavirus in infants: Relationships between infection rate and mode of delivery." *Obstetrics and Gynecology* 91, no. 1 (January): 92–96.

Villa, L. L. 2000. "Critical view on HPV detection methods." Paper presented at the 18th International Papillomavirus Conference and HPV Clinical Workshop jointly with the 12th Meeting of the AEPCC, Barcelona, Spain, July.

von Krogh, G., C.J.N. Lacey, G. Gross, R. Barrasso, and A. Schneider. 2000. "Guidelines for primary care physicians for the diagnosis and management of anogenital warts." Paper presented at the 18th International Papillomavirus Conference and HPV Clinical Workshop jointly with the 12th Meeting of the AEPCC, Barcelona, Spain, July.

Zarcone, R., G. Mainini, E. Carfora, and A. Cardone. 1997. "Current etiopathogenetic views in vulvar cancer." *Panminerva Medica* 39, no. 1 (March): 30–34.

INTERNET SOURCES

"Anal cancer PDQ." 1999.
*www.cancer.gov/cancer_information/menu_multi.aspx?viewid=
d3d92ba5-9709-454c-bb12-5ee5ded7c7bb*

"Cervical cancer PDQ." September 2000.
*www.cancer.gov/cancer_information/doc_pdq.aspx?version=pati
ent&viewid=862ac265-8ff9-4bc5-8b68-1458c603548d*

"Cervical dysplasia: Nutrition and dietary supplements."
*www.ivillagehealth.com/library/onemed/content/0,7064,241012
_245583,00.html#nutritiondiet*

"Chemotherapy and you." June 1999.
www.cancer.gov/cancer_information/doc_img.aspx?viewid=d74
    c07e0-0539-4253-b700-87c1eb162b09

Cornforth, Tracee. "Vaginal yeast infections." October 1998.
http://womenshealth.about.com/library/weekly/aa102298.htm

———. "Bacterial vaginosis." January 1999.
http://womenshealth.about.com/library/weekly/aa010199.htm

———. "Genital herpes." November 1999.
http://womenshealth.about.com/library/weekly/aa112399.htm

———. "Trichomonas, trichomoniasis, trich." December 1999.
http://womenshealth.about.com/library/weekly/aa120799a.htm

Jelovsek, F. R. "Abnormal Pap smear with atypical squamous
    cell changes: ASCUS."
http://www.wdxcyber.com/npapvg13.htm

———. "Natural progression of an abnormal Pap."
http://www.wdxcyber.com/npapvg08.htm

———. "What to expect after hysterectomy."
http://www.wdxcyber.com/nbleed13.htm

"Penile cancer PDQ." 1999.
www.cancer.gov/cancer_information/doc_pdq.aspx?viewid=A68
    3F65E-43B1-4226-AC56-97E56512F666

"Radiation therapy and you." September 1999.
www.cancer.gov/cancer_information/doc_img.aspx?viewid=321
    36103-0800-407b-83c8-28fd87267753

"Vulvar cancer PDQ." 1999.
www.cancer.gov/cancer_information/menu_multi.aspx?viewid=
709f2d27-e92f-4f8d-aace-66935e8dde0f

"What you need to know about cancer of the cervix."
September 1998.
www.cancer.gov/cancer_information/doc_wyntk.aspx?viewid=15
2972f-0309-4f59-aa5f-a17a761f10d9

INDEX

Note: Page numbers in italics refers to illustrations

abdominoperineal resection, 242, 245
acetowhitening, 99, 258
acetylsalicylic acid (ASA), 134
acyclovir, *see* Zovirax (acyclovir)
adenocarcinoma:
   of the cervix, 54–55, 111–12
   vaginal, 186, 188
African-American women, cervical
      cancer among, 146
age:
   HPV, cervical dysplasia, and cervical
      cancer, 17–19, *18,* 46, 47–48, 125
   vaginal cancer and, 186–87, 201
   vulvar dysplasia and vulvar cancer
      and, 204, 213
AIN (anal intraepithelial neoplasia), *see*
      anal dysplasia
alopecia (hair loss), as chemotherapy
      side effect, 170–71
American Cancer Society, 63, 153
American College of Obstetrics and
      Gynecology, 63
American Medical Association, 291
American Social Health Association, xi
amino acids, 13
anal cancer, xii, 239–49
   incidence of, 218
   prevention of, 246
   recurrent, 243
   staging of, 241
      treatment and, 241–43
   symptoms of, 240

   treatment of, 241–46
   staging and, 241–43
anal dysplasia, 219, 222–39
   abnormal anal pap smear, responding
      to, 227–30
   anal pap smear, 225–27
   candidates for screening, 223–25
   high-risk women and, 222, 224
   in men, 312–16
   prevention of, 246
   risk factors for, 247
   severe, *231*
      treatment of, 233–39
   symptoms of, 222–23
   talking to your doctor about, 248–49
   treatment of, 230–39
      mild dysplasia, 232–33
      moderate and severe dysplasia,
         233–39
anal HPV infection, 219–21
anal incontinence, 232, 238
anal intraepithelial neoplasia (AIN), *see*
      anal dysplasia
anal-oral sex, 336
anal Pap smear, 225–27
anal sex, 42, 215–17, 247, 317
   men who have sex with men (MSM),
      313–14, 315
anorectal junction, 239, 240
anorexia, 126
antibiotics, yeast infections and, 83, 85
antibodies, 344

antioxidants, 126–27
antiviral medicines for HPV, 349
anus:
    genital warts in anal canal, 262–63,
        266
    perianal area, 216, 222, 234, 239
        genital warts of, 262–63, 266, 297
    transformation zone (TZ), 219, *220,*
        231
ASCUS diagnosis, Pap smear with, *see*
        Pap smears, ASCUS (atypical
        squamous cell changes of
        undetermined significance)
        diagnosis
aspirin, 134
Astruc, John, 10
AutoPap 300 QC, 70–71

bacterial vaginosis, 85–87, 97
benzodiazepines, 238
Bethesda system, *see* Pap smears,
        Bethesda system
bichloracetic acid, 267
biopsy:
    cervical, 58–59, *59*
        classification systems, 27–29, *28*
    colposcopy, *see* colposcopy
    cone, *see* cone biopsy (conization)
    Pap smear distinguished from, 27
    of penile lesions, 296, 299–300
birth control pills, 45, 46, 84, 125
bleomycin, 310
blood tests, 152
B lymphocytes, 344
Bosanquet, N., 71
bowenoid papulosis, 304–305, *306*
Bowen's disease, *223,* 234
Boxman, I. L., 261
bulimia, 126

Campion, M. J., 10, 258
Cancer Information service, 153
candida albicans, 83, 97
carcinoma in situ, *16,* 118, 153–54, 208,
        242
CD4 lymphocytes, 314
Centers for Disease Control and
        Prevention, 268
cervical cancer, 24, 32–37, *58, 59,*
        146–81
    adenocarcinoma, 54–55, 111–12

age-related prevalence of, *18,* 48–49
among African-American women, 146
diagnosis of, 149–50
fertility and, 178–79
metastasis of, 148
oncogenic forms of HPV and, 10
Pap smears to detect, *see* Pap smears
precancerous cervical disease, *see*
        cervical dysplasia
pregnancy and, 179–80
screening for, *see* Pap smears
staging of, 151–53
    treatment according to, 153–56
statistics, xi–xii, 10, 56, 146
support groups, 180–81
survival rate, 147, 152
symptoms of, 148
treatment options:
    chemotherapy, 154–56, 167–73
    clinical trials, 153, 156, 173–77
    external radiation therapy, 154–56,
        164–67
    hysterectomy, 154, 156–61
    internal radiation therapy, 154–56,
        161–64
    by stage, 153–56
cervical cytology, *see* Pap smears
cervical dysplasia, 4, 24, 30–37, 336
    age-related prevalence of, *18,* 47–49
    biopsy classification systems, 27–29, *28*
    discussing with your doctor, 128
    immunosuppression and, 122–23
    mild, *16, 18, 28,* 29–30, 31, 48, 55,
        57, 59, 108, 115–28
        biopsy of, *25*
        pregnancy and, 122
        treatment of, 121–22
    moderate and severe, *16, 28,* 29,
        30–31, 48, 55, *57, 59,* 108, 118
        fertility and, 140–41
        pregnancy and, 141–42
        prevention of future, 142–43
        rate of progress of, 131–32
        talking to your doctor, 144–45
        treatment methods, 133–40, 141
    Pap smears, *see* Pap smears
    risk factors for, 40–41, 45–46, 124–26
    sexual partners, discussion with, 143
cervical incompetence, 52
cervical intraepithelial neoplasia, *see*
        cervical dysplasia

cervical stenosis, 135
cervicitis, 85–87
cervix, 52–55, 57
    anatomy, 52–53, *53*
    cervical cancer, *see* cervical cancer
    cervical dysplasia, *see* cervical
        dysplasia
    endocervical columnar epithelium of,
        19–20, 53–54, 57
    epithelium of the, 14–22, 52–55
    exocervical squamous epithelium of,
        19–20, 53–54, 57
    functions of, 52
    genital warts of the, *see* genital warts,
        cervical
    normal, *57, 58, 59*
    polyps and cysts of the, 147
    self-exam, 367
    transformation zone (TZ), 19–20, *20,*
        53–54, 57, 136, *220,* 256
cesarean birth, 280, 281
chemotherapy:
    for anal cancer, 243, 244–45
    for cervical cancer, 154–56, 167–73
    coping with, 172–73
    for penile cancer, 310, 311, 312
    side effects of, 169–72, 178
    support groups, 172–73
    for vaginal cancer, 198
    for vulvar cancer, 209
childbirth, HPV transmitted at, *see*
        recurrent respiratory
        papillomatosis (RRP)
cidofovir, 284
circumcision for penile cancer, 309, 312
cisplatin-based drugs, 167–68, 245, 310
Cleocin 2, 86
clinical trials:
    for anal cancer, 245–46
    becoming involved in, 175–76
    for cervical cancer, 153, 156, 173–77
    informed consent for, 175–76
    for penile cancer, 312
    phases of, 174
    talking to your doctor about
        participation in, 176–77
    types of, 173–74
    for vaginal cancer, 198, 199, 200
    for vulvar cancer, 212
"cold-knife" conization, *see* cone biopsy
    (conization)

cold-scapel excision, 191–92
colon cancer, 239–40
colonization, 280
colonoscopy, 240
colostomy, 242, 245
colposcope, *100,* 139, 294
colposcopy, 105, 149
    after abnormal Pap smear, 58–62, 154
        AGUS diagnosis, 112
        ASCUS diagnosis, 96, 98–101, 110
        HSIL diagnosis, 130, 141
        LSIL diagnosis, 119
    cervical cancer diagnosed with, 150
    genital warts viewed during, 256, 257,
        258
    for penile cancer, 308, 316
    for vaginal dysplasia, 189–90
    for vulvar dysplasia, 205–206
communication with sexual partners, *see*
        sexual partners, communication
        with
computerized tomography (CT) (CAT
        scan), 152
condoms, 84, 94
    for anal intercourse, 246
    HPV transmission, to reduce, xiii,
        39–40, 44–45, 304, 317, 331–32,
        338
    incomplete protection of penis from
        HPV infection, 290–91
    STD prevention and, 85, 90, 91, 93
condyloma acuminata, *see* genital warts
condylomata latum, 296
cone biopsy (conization), 102, 112,
    137–38, *138,* 141, 142, 154
    cervical cancer diagnosed with, 150
Covens, A. P., 178
cryotherapy, 138–39, 141, 194–95, 206,
    232, 234, 257, 259, 267, 272, 303,
    306, 335
cystoscopy, 152
cytopathologist, 57, 62, 67
cytotechnologist, 57, 61–62, 67–68, 71
Cytyc Corporation, 70

DES (diethylstilbestrol), vaginal
        adenocarcinomas and, 186, 188,
        201
diabetes, 83–84, 86
diagnosis, *see specific conditions*
diet, *see* nutrition

diethylstilbestrol (DES), vaginal
    adenocarcinomas and, 186, 188,
    201
Diflucan, 84
dilation and curettage (D&C), 102–103
DNA, 11–14, *25*
  E6, E7, p53 and pRB proteins and
    damage to, *34,* 35–36
doctors, 81
  relationship with, 81–82
  talking to your:
    about anal dysplasia, 248–49
    about ASCUS diagnosis of Pap
      smear, 113–14
    about clinical trial participation,
      176–77
    about genital warts, 264–65
    about HPV, 50
    about LSIL diagnosis of Pap smear,
      128
    about mild cervical dysplasia, 128
    about moderate to severe cervical
      dysplasia, 144–45
    about Pap smears, 81, 94, 113–14,
      128
    about STDs, 4–5
douching, 85, 93
dysplasia, *see specific locations of
    dysplasia, e.g.* cervical dysplasia

Efudex, *see* 5-fluorouracil (Efudex)
Elamax-5, 238
El-Bastawissi, A. Y., 141
electrical wire loop electrode, *61,* 134
electrocautery, 237, 273
electrodessication, 273
electrosurgery, 306
endocervical curettage (ECC), 101–102,
    257
epithelium, 6–8
  basal cells, 15, 17, 19, 21, 24–25
  basement membrane, 14, *16,* 147
  cutaneous, 6–7, 8
  HPV life cycle and, 14–22
  mucosal, 6–7, 8
  stroma, 14, *16*
exercise, 246

family history of cervical cancer, 45, 125
Famvir (famcyclovir), 89
fertility:

cervical cancer and, 178–79
chemotherapy and, 172, 178
moderate or severe cervical dysplasia
    and, 140–41
radiation therapy and, 164, 178
5-fluorouracil (Efudex), 140, 168, 169,
    171, 244, 245, 257, 303, 310
  cream, 193–94, 206, 275, 309
Flagyl (metronidazole), 86, 91
folic acid, 126, 127, 349
Food and Drug Administration, 103
forceps, biopsy, *60,* 101
future developments for HPV
    prevention and treatment, 343–50
  antiviral medicines, 349
  vaccines, 343–49
    prophylactic, 344–47
    therapeutic, 344–45, 347–49

Gardnerella vaginalis, 86
genes, 12
  oncogenes, 32
  tumor suppressors, 33
genetics:
  immune response and, 21–22
genital warts, 10–11, 121, 253–78, 333
  in anal canal, 262–63, 266
  as benign tumors, 147
  cervical, 23–26, 255–57
    diagnosis of, 256
    symptoms of, 256–57
    treatment of, 257
  clinical significance of, 255
  contagion of HPV and, 26, 37, 255,
    256
  HPV types causing, 9, 24, 254
  living with, 336
  men and, 266–67
  perianal, 262–63, 266
  recurrence of, 261, 277, 336
  risk factors for, 263
  talking to your doctor about, 264–65
  treatment of, 266–78
    chart, 269
    follow-up, 277
    patient-applied, 267, 268–71
    provider-administered, 267, 271–76
    vaginal, 257–59
    vulvar, 259–61, *260,* 266
genome, 12, 14
  HPV, *13,* 14

glossary, 351–62
Groopman, Dr. Jerome, 149
gynecologic oncologist, 153
gynecologist, choosing your, 363–64

herpes simplex virus (HSV), 17, 87–90
highly active antiretroviral therapy
(HAART), 314–15, 316
high-resolution anoscopy (HRA),
228–30, 232, 240, 315
HIV (human immunodeficiency virus),
3, 19, 39, 46, 123, 125, 201, 213,
221, 224, 261, 304, 307, 314–16
hoarseness, 282, 283
homosexuality, *see* MSM (men who
have sex with men); WSW
(women who have sex with
women)
hormone replacement therapy, 157, 160
radical, with lymph node dissection,
154, 157
HPV (human papillomavirus), xii
age-related prevalence of, 17–19, *18,*
47–49, 125
anal cancer and, *see* anal cancer
anal infection, 219–21
benign infections:
genital warts, *see* genital warts
recurrent respiratory papillomatosis,
279–85
benign (nononcogenic) types, 8, 21
HPV 6 and 11, 8, 9, 24, 119,
253–54, 262, 263, 284, 349
cancer causing forms of, *see this entry*
under oncogenic types
cervical cancer and, *see* cervical
cancer
common questions of people infected
with, 321–39
communication with sexual partners,
see sexual partners,
communication with
condom use, *see* condoms
dormant, 19, 21
E6 and E7 proteins, 30, 32–37, *34,*
132, 347–48
the future, *see* future developments
for HPV prevention and
treatment
incubation period, 23, 143, 323

infection of the epithelium, *see*
epithelium
life changes after diagnosis with, 336
life cycle of, 14–22
men and, *see* men and HPV
oncogenic types, xiv, 8, 9–10, 21
HPV 16 and 18, 8, 9, 14, 24, 55,
254
HPV 16 and 19, 349
p53 and pRB cellular proteins, 32–37,
34, 132
penile cancer and, *see* penile cancer
recurrence of, 333–34
risk factors for, 47–49, *see* risk factors,
for HPV
sexual partners and, *see* sexual
partners
statistics, xii–xiii, 3
support groups, 336
test for, *see* Hybrid Capture II (HC-II)
test
transmission by skin-to-skin contact,
xiii, 7, 8, 39, 41–44, 290–91
periods of greatest contagion, 26,
37–39
types of, 6–8, 21, 253–54
chart, 9
variants, 132
vaginal cancer and, *see* vaginal cancer
virology and, 11–14
vulvar cancer and, *see* vulvar cancer
who infected you, trying to
determine, 323–24
HRA, *see* high-resolution anoscopy
(HRA)
HSIL (high-grade squamous
intraepithelial lesion), *see* Pap
smears, HSIL (high-grade
squamous intraepithelial lesion)
diagnosis
Human Genome Project, 14
human papillomavirus (HPV), *see* HPV
(human papillomavirus)
Hybrid Capture II (HC-II) test, 63, 96,
98, 103–109, 230
ASCUS diagnosis on Pap smear and,
103–106
hydrocortisone cream, 298
hygiene, 93, 263
hyperkeratotic warts, 255
hysterectomy, 140

hysterectomy (*cont.*)
  for cervical cancer, 154, 156–61
  postoperative care, 158–60
  the procedure, 157–58
  support groups, 160–61
  total, 157
  total abdominal, with bilateral salpingo-oophorectomy (TAH-BSO), 157
  for vaginal cancer, 197, 200

ibuprofen, 134
imiquimod, 267, 271, 303, 349
immune response, 21–22, 45, 46, 47, 48, 86, 93–94, 110, 125, 143, 263, 285, 307
  anal dysplasia and, 247
  cell-mediated immune system, 344, 345
  cervical dysplasia and immunosuppression, 122–23
  genital warts and, 255, 257
  humoral immune system, 344, 345
  pregnancy and, *see* pregnancy, immunity during
immunosuppressants, 110
indole-3 carbinol, 284, 349
informed consent for clinical trial participation, 175–76
infrared coagulation (IRC), 233
interferon therapy, 267, 275–76
International AIDS Conference, 2000, xiii

Kaposi's sarcoma, 314
Kashima, H. K., 283
keratin, 6, 255
kidney transplants, 123
koilocytes, *16*, 25–26, 255
koilocytosis, 26

lactobacilli, 83, 86
Lamb, H. M., 271
laparoscopy, 178–79
large loop excision of the transformation zone (LLETZ), *see* LEEP (loop electrosurgical excision procedure)
laser ablation, 239
laser conization, 139–40
laser therapy, 257

carbon dioxide, 275, 284
  for vaginal dysplasia, 191–92
  for vulvar dysplasia, 206
laser vaporization, 259, 306
LEEP (loop electrosurgical excision procedure), *61,* 112, 154, 257, 336
  for anal dysplasia, 231
  for moderate to severe cervical dysplasia, 133–36, 142
  for vaginal dysplasia, 191
lichen planus, 298
lichen sclerosis, 213
lidocaine, 238
liquid nitrogen therapy, *see* cryotherapy
LLETZ (large loop excision of the transformation zone), *see* LEEP (loop electrosurgical excision procedure)
loop electrosurgical excision procedure, *see* LEEP (loop electrosurgical excision procedure)
LSIL (low-squamous intraepithelial lesions), *see* Pap smears, LSIL (low-squamous intraepithelial lesions) diagnosis
Lugol's solution, 101
lymph nodes, 148, 152, 197, 208, 209, 242, 243
  dissection, 243, 245

Meirow, D., 179
men and HPV, 289–317
  anal HPV infection and anal dysplasia, 312–16
  penis, *see* penis
menopause, 86
  chemotherapy and, 172
  surgical, 160
men who have sex with men, *see* MSM (men who have sex with men)
metastasis, 7, 147–48
  of cervical cancer, 148
  of vaginal cancer, 187
methotrexate, 310
metronidazole, *see* Flagyl (metronidazole)
microlaryngoscopy, 284
microsurgery for penile cancer, 309–11
Miller, A. B., 56
mitomycin C, 244

Mounts, P., 283
mouth:
  cancer of the, xii
  HPV types affecting the, 8
  oral cancers, 335
MSM (men who have sex with men):
  anal cancer and, 218
  anal HPV infection and anal
    dysplasia, 313–14
  screening for anal dysplasia, 224
mucous membranes, 6

National Cancer Institute, 153, 175,
    176
National Institutes of Health, 175
New Yorker, The, 149, 152
nonoxynol-9, 349
nutrition, 22, 46, 94, 110, 125, 126–27,
    143, 246, 304, 337
  during chemotherapy, 171

obesity, 46, 84, 125
"Of Porri, Verrucae and Condylomata of
    the Pudenda," 10–11
oncogenes, 32
oncogenic types of HPV, *see* HPV
    (human papillomavirus),
    oncogenic types
"On Warty Excrescences of the Female
    Genitalia," 10
oral-anal sex, 336
oral contraceptives, *see* birth control
    pills
oral sex, 43, 89, 334–35
organ transplants, immunosuppression
    and, 122–23

palliative treatment, 156, 198, 209, 243
Papanicolaou, George, 10, 56
papillary lesion, 100
PAPNET, 70–71
Pap smears, xii, 51–145, 152, 189,
    337–38
  abnormal, 317
    ASCUS diagnosis, *see this entry*
      under ASCUS diagnosis
    attitude toward, 95–96, 150
    HSIL diagnosis, *see this entry under*
      HSIL (high-grade squamous
      intraepithelial lesion) diagnosis
  accuracy of, 64–66

AGUS diagnosis, 111–12
anal, 225–27, 315
ASCUS (atypical squamous cell
    changes of undetermined
    significance) diagnosis, *28,*
    95–114, 150
  ASC-H (cells that cannot exclude
    HSIL), 96, 98
  ASC-US (unsatisfactory
    significance), 96, 98
  discussion with your doctor,
    113–14
  follow-up options, 96, 98–109, 110
  meaning of, 96–98
  pregnancy and, 110–11
  recurrent, 109–10
  regression to normal, 97–98
  statistics, *97*
"benign cellular changes," 82–92, 94
Bethesda system, 27–28, *28,* 29,
    62–63, 96, *116–17*
  biopsy distinguished from, 27
  class system, 27–*28,* 62
  computerized screening of cervical
    smears, 70–71
  false negatives, 65, 67, 68
  false positives, 68–69, 105
  follow-up test for abnormal, *see*
    colposcopy
  frequency, 63–64, 73, 82
  HPV test distinguished from, 63
  HSIL (high-grade squamous
    intraepithelial lesion) diagnosis,
    28, 97, 129–45, *132,* 149
  incorrect results, 66–69
  invention of, 10
  LSIL (low-squamous intraepithelial
    lesions) diagnosis, *28, 97,*
    114–28, *116–17,* 149
    follow-up treatment, 118–19
    meaning of, 117–20
    newer methods of performing,
      69–73
  newer methods of performing:
    ThinPrep test, 70, 104, 106
  Polarprobe, 71–73
  pregnancy and, 122
  preparing for, 66–67, 80
  the procedure, 56–58, 60–62
  recommendation for screening, 73–75
  role of, 59, 121

Pap smears (*cont.*)
  symptoms of, 120–21
  talking to your doctor, 81, 94, 128
  treatment of, 121–22
  "unsatisfactory rating," 79–80, 94
  "within normal limits," 80–82, 94
pelvic examination, 60, 152, 189, 205
  self-exam, 365–67
pelvic exenteration, 198–99, 200, 209, 212
pelvic inflammatory disease (PID), 85
penectomy, 310, 311, 312
penile cancer, xii, 290, 306, 308–312
  incidence of, 291
  staging and treatment of, 309–12
  symptoms of, 308
penile dysplasia (penile intraepithelial neoplasia), 296, 304–307, *306,* 308
penis, 289–312, *295*
  cancer of, *see* penile cancer
  circumcision for penile cancer, 309, 312
  circumcised men and HPV, 290, 308
  condom use, incomplete protection against HPV by, 290–91
  diagnosis of diseases of the, 298–99
  examination of, 291–93, 293–97
  frenulum, *295,* 296
  HPV testing and, 290, 300–301
  lesions, diagnosis of, 299–300
  pearly penile papules, *295,* 295–96
  self-exam, 299, 368–69
  subclinical infections, 291, 298
  Tyson's glands, *295,* 296
  uncircumcized men and HPV, 290, 307
  "vinegar" test with magnification, 291, 301, 316
  warts on the, 301–304, *302*
perfumed products, 94
Perry, C. M., 271
Phelps, W. C., 349
physicians, *see* doctors
podofilox, 267, 270, 303
podophyllin resin, 267, 274, 335
Polarprobe, 71–73
pregnancy:
  ASCUS diagnosis on Pap smear and, 110–11
  cervical cancer and, 179–80
  chemotherapy during, 172

genital herpes simplex virus and, 90
genital wart treatments and, 268, 270, 274, 276
immunity during, 84, 110–11, 125, 257, 261
mild dysplasia and, 122
moderate or severe cervical dysplasia, 141–42
radiation therapy during, 164
proctosigmoidoscopy, 152
prostate gland, 216
protease inhibitors, 314
pruritis, 258
psoriasis, 298

radiation proctitis, 244
radiation therapy:
  for anal cancer, 242, 243, 244
  external, 154–56, 164–67, 197–98, 199, 310
  fertility and, 164, 178
  internal (intracaviary), 154–56, 161–64, 197–98, 199
  for penile cancer, 310, 311, 312
  recurrent respiratory papillomatosis and, 285
  for vulvar cancer, 208, 209, 211
radical local excision and groin lymph node removal, 208, 211
radical vulvectomy with lymph node dissection, 208–209, 211
rectal cancer, 239–40
Recurrent Respiratory Papillomatosis Foundation, 285
recurrent respiratory papillomatosis (RRP), 279–85, 349
  adult-onset, 281, 283
  juvenile-onset, 281, 282–83
  risk factors for, 284–85
  support groups for, 285
  transmission of, 281–82
  treatment of, 284
resources, 370–72
retinoic acid, 140, 349
retractor, 237
risk factors:
  for dysplasia, 40–41, 45–46, 124–26
  for genital warts, 263
  for HPV, 21–22, 40–45, 124
    see also smoking; *specific factors, e.g.* nutrition

for recurrent respiratory
    papillomatosis (RRP), 284–85
for vaginal cancer, 201
for vulvar cancer, 213
RNA, 11–12
Ronnett, B. M., 112
RRP, *see* recurrent respiratory
    papillomatosis (RRP)

second opinions, 153
self-exam:
    cervical, 367
    pelvic, 365–67
    of the penis, 299, 368–69
    vaginal, 200–201, 258, 367
    vulvar, 212, 366
sexually transmitted diseases (STDs), 4,
    263
    condoms to prevent, *see* condoms,
        STD prevention and
    emotional toll of, 321–22
    history of, 45, 124, 307
    HPV, *see* HPV (human
        papillomavirus)
    three Cs for avoiding, 93
sexual partners:
    care in choosing, 5, 317, 338
    communication with, 39–40, 93,
        321–30
        about cervical dysplasia, 143
        current partner, 324–25
        future partners, 328–30
        previous partner(s), 326–28
    multiple, 44, 47
    reinfection by, 333–34
    screening male partners of women
        with HPV, 293, 317
    testing for HPV, 332–33
Shah, K. V., 32, 283
shaving of pubic hair, 261, 306
Singer, A., 71, 72
sitz baths, 238, 239, 244
skinning vulvectomy, 206, 210–11
smoking, 22, 36, 45, 94, 110, 124, 126,
        132, 143, 201, 213, 246, 247,
        255, 263, 285, 304, 307, 337
socioeconomic status as risk factor,
        213
    for cervical dysplasia, 46, 125
    for vaginal cancer, 201
speculum, vaginal, 60, 61, 99, 100

squamous intraepithelial lesions (SIL),
    29
staging, *see specific forms of cancer*
stenosis, 232, 238
stress, 22, 45, 124, 126, 333–34
subclinical infection, 23, 37, 121, 223,
    291, 304
support groups, 372
    cervical cancer, 180–81
    for chemotherapy patients, 172–73
    HPV, 336
    hysterectomy, 160–61
    for recurrent respiratory
        papillomatosis (RRP), 285
surgical excision:
    for anal dysplasia, 236–38
    of genital warts, 275
    of oral cancers, 335
syphilis, secondary, 296

TCA (trichloroacetic acid):
    for anal dysplasia, 232, 234
    for genital warts, 257, 267, 272–73
    for penile dysplasia, 306
    for penile warts, 303
    for vulvar dysplasia, 206
    for vaginal dysplasia, 195–96
T-helper lymphocytes, 314
ThinPrep test, 70, 104, 106
T lymphocytes, 344, 348
trachelectomy, 154, 178
treatment, *see specific conditions*
trichomonas infection, 91, 97
tumors:
    benign, 147
    malignant, 147–48

underwear, cotton, 84, 85, 87, 91, 93
urinary tract infections, 217
urine analysis, 152
uterus, 53

vaccines against HPV, 343, 344–49
    prophylactic, 344–47
    therapeutic, 344–45, 347–49
vagina, 53, 185
    construction of new, 197, 199, 200
    genital warts of the, 257–59
    self-exam, 200–201, 258, 367
vaginal cancer, xii, 185–88, 196–202
    adenocarcinomas, 186, 188, 201

vaginal cancer (*cont.*)
  incidence of, 186
  metastasis of, 187
  recurrent, 198–99
  risk factors for, 201
  self-exam, 200–201, 258, 367
  squamous cell, 186–87, 201
  staging of, 196
    treatment and, 197–98
  treatment of, 197–200
    staging and, 197–98
vaginal dysplasia, 188–96
  diagnosis of, 189–90
  other name for, 187
  staging of, 190–91
  symptoms of, 189
  treatment of, 191–96
vaginal intraepithelial neoplasia (VAIN),
    see vaginal dysplasia
vaginectomy, 197, 199, 200
VAIN (vaginal intraepithelial neoplasia),
    see vaginal dysplasia
Valtrex (valacyclovir), 89
vascular mosaicism, 100
vascular punctation, 100
vincristine, 310
VIN (vulvar intraepithelial neoplasia),
    see vulvar dysplasia
virology of HPV, 11–14
vitamin A, 349
vitamin C, 126, 127
vitamin E, 126, 127
vitamin supplements, 127
vulva, *53,* 203
  genital warts of the, 259–61, *260,*
    266

  parts of the, 203–204
  self-exam, 212, 366
vulvar cancer, xii, 203–14
  age and, 204, 213
  rarity of, 203
  recurrent, 209
  risk factors for, 213
  self-exam, 212, 366
  staging of, 207
    treatment and, 208–209
  survival rates, 207
  symptoms of, 204–205
  treatment of, 208–12
    staging and, 208–209
vulvar dysplasia, 188, 203–206, 214
  age and, 204
  diagnosis of, 205–206
  staging and treatment of, 206
  symptoms of, 204–205
vulvar intraepithelial neoplasia (VIN),
    see vulvar dysplasia

warts, HPV-caused, 4, 7, 8, 23
  genital, *see* genital warts
  palmar and plantar, 7–8, 254
  on the penis, 301–304, *302*
wide local excision, 197, 199, 200, 206,
    208, 210, 309, 311
WSW (women who have sex with
    women), Pap smears and, 64

x-rays, 152

yeast infections, 82–85, 298

Zovirax (acyclovir), 89

ABOUT THE AUTHOR

Dr. Palefsky is a professor of medicine at the University of California, San Francisco. He trained in internal medicine at McGill Univerity in Montreal, Canada, and in infectious diseases at Stanford University. An internationally known expert on human papillomaviruses and the diseases that they cause in men and women, he has published over one hundred articles and book chapters on HPV.